Release Your
Shoulders,
Relax Your
Neck

The best exercises for relieving tight shoulders & neck pain.

Howard VanEs, M.A. ERYT-500

Letsdoyoga.com Wellness Series

Copyright 2012, by Howard Allan VanEs and Letsdoyoga.com. All rights reserved. Except as permitted under the United States Copyright Act of 1976, no part of this publication may be reproduced or distributed in any form or by any means without prior written consent of the publisher.

Published by
Letsdoyoga.com

Howard VanEs, publisher
4651 Antelope Way
Antioch CA 94531
www.letsdoyoga.com
info@letsdoyoga.com

Disclaimer

The information in this booklet is not intended to diagnose or treat any health condition and is for educational purposes. If you are experiencing any pain, numbness, stiffness, weakness or any other symptom in any part of your body it is highly advisable to seek the advice of a physician or qualified health care practitioner.

Free Wellness Newsletter

As a service to our readers Letsdoyoga.com publishes a wellness newsletter. This monthly newsletter features articles and ideas to help you live a happier and healthier life as well as insights, tips and ideas to deepen the practice of yoga. If you would like to receive a copy of Yoga Health and Wellness Newsletter visit **www.letsdoyoga.com** and enter your email address.

Acknowledgements

Letsdoyoga.com would like to acknowledge and thank the following people whose contribution was integral to the production of this book:

Designer: Howard Petlack, hpetlack@agoodthingink.com

Photographer: Karen Margroff Dunn, KMDPortraits.com

Models: Lois Kaye Pope and Gary Martin
Contact them in care of info@letsdoyoga.com

Location: The Yoga and Movement Center, Walnut Creek, CA
Diane Valentine, Director, www.yoga-movement.com

Letsdoyoga.com offers seminars and workshops on the following wellness related topics:

Stress management

Office ergonomics

Insomnia

Anxiety

Tight shoulders

Back care

Abdominal exercises

Meditation

Pranayama (yogic breathing)

Secrets of stretching

Various Yoga oriented workshops

If you are interested in have any of the above trainings presented to your organization please contact Howard VanEs at **info@letsdoyoga.com** or 415-309-1290.

Table of Contents

Introduction   *7*

About The Author   *9*

About Your Tight Shoulders & Neck   *11*

Shoulder Anatomy 101   *19*

Shoulder Muscles   *22*

Shoulder Joint   *24*

Before You Begin—How to Use This Book   *25*

How Breathing Affects Your Shoulders & Neck   *29*

Exercises   *33*

Additional Ideas of Interest   *85*

Publications of Interest   *91*

Introduction

By Rick Harvey, Doctor of Chiropractic

Do you have pain or tightness in your shoulders? There is a good chance that you do. The shoulder is the most mobile joint in the human body and this flexibility comes at a price: increased risk of injury. Shoulder injuries develop over time from repetitive strain or acutely from a sudden fall or accident. The care and management of the shoulder must be addressed in a logical and well thought out manner.

These injuries can and do affect people of all ages from those in elementary school to college to those who are middle aged as well as seniors; athlete or non-athlete are all vulnerable. Regardless of gender, working individuals who spend their days at the computer, driving trucks or even taking care of children are all subject to the injury prone shoulder. The weekend athlete, tennis or soccer player and even the dart thrower can be just waiting for the tiny "catch" and sharp pain that stops all activity and disrupts their life. Even those in their golden years do not seem to be immune from the all-vulnerable shoulder. Conservative treatment for shoulder injuries can include medication, physical therapy and finally, surgery.

As you now realize, the shoulder injury is here to stay. The questions then become: Why is the shoulder so injury prone? What can I do to prevent injuring my shoulder? What can I do if I have already injured my shoulder?

As a practicing Doctor of Chiropractic for almost 30 years, I have had the opportunity to treat thousands of individuals with either acute and/or chronic shoulder problems. I have seen injuries from activities as simple as a fall in the garden, throwing a baseball a little too hard, to sleeping with the arm in the wrong position to something more serious, such as a head-on auto accident. Most, if not all of these problems could have been prevented and assisted in their recovery if only a few simple steps had been taken. The understanding of the shoulder is something even those of us with years of experience in diagnosing and managing/treating find difficult to treat. I have consulted numerous sources and spent significant time explaining the shoulder and its treatment protocol in detail to my patients.

Howard presents a much needed and well thought out text to this most versatile and complex joint. He provides you with a simple but comprehensive understanding of the anatomy of this joint and how it works. By providing us with a series of excellent exercises and stretching activities he has given us with a logical approach to help us in preventing shoulder injuries as well as relief for those who are experiencing tight shoulders or limited range of motion. I continue to refer to this useful resource in ongoing treatment of my patients and highly recommend that those who are experiencing shoulder and neck issues order a copy.

Dr. Richard S Harvey
Doctor of Chiropractic
18080 San Ranon Valley Blvd.
San Ramon, CA 94583
dr.rick47@comcast.net

About the Author

Howard VanEs, M.A., ERYT-500, has been committed to wellness and fitness for over 25 years. He has a deep passion for wellness, and a desire to help people learn about the many ways they can improve the quality of their health and lives through mind/body methods. His experience includes weight training, martial arts, yoga, stress management training, and work from his previous role as a psychotherapist. For over 20 years, Howard has been a dedicated practitioner of hatha yoga and has been teaching yoga for the last 15 years in the Bay Area of California.

Howard is the author of *Ageless Beauty & Timeless Strength, Meditation: The Gift Inside How to meditate to quiet your mind, find inner peace and lasting happiness* and is the primary author and editor of the Letsdoyoga.com wellness book series: *Beginning Yoga: A Practice Manual, Abs!, Tight Shoulder Relief* and co-author of *Office Ergonomics, Preventing Repetitive Motion Injuries and Carpal Tunnel Syndrome*. He is also the co-producer of the audio CD, *Shavasna/Deep Relaxation*, and creator of the *Yoga on Demand* audio program which features over 14 yoga audios. In addition to writing about and teaching yoga, Howard also leads yoga teacher trainings, wellness seminars and retreats worldwide.

His websites are:

www.letsdoyoga.com
www.exercisesforupperbody.com
www.agelessbeautybook.com
www.yogameditationinstruction.com

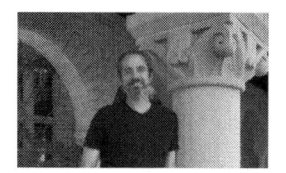

About Your Tight Shoulders

If you are reading this book chances are good that either you or someone you know has a shoulder issue. In fact, according to the National Center for Health Studies approximately 13.7 million people visited a doctor in 2003 for a shoulder problem. And those are just statistics for people who have seen a doctor. It doesn't include those have shoulder problems but haven't seen a doctor! What's more, many health experts suggest that most people will have some sort of shoulder issues by the time they reach 65 years of age.

So, what leads to tight shoulders and shoulder related injuries? The answer is that are many factors contributing to this - some of which that are preventable and others that are not.

A major factor is your career choice—what you are doing on a day to day basis. If you are involved in a job which requires a lot of repetitive motions then you are at risk. People who spend a lot of time working on computers, dental hygienists, gardeners, hair stylists, and professional athletes are examples of professions where there is a high prevalence of shoulder issues from overuse.

Stress and emotions contribute to tight shoulders as well. Many people carry stress in their shoulders. Prior and current injuries to your shoulder also directly impact how well they function as well as any past surgery, illness or disease such as arthritis, bursitis, bone spurs, etc. Another contributing factor to be considered is your genetics: your posture, how well your body handles stress and the inherent strength or weakness of your muscles and connective tissues. Your general fitness level and your diet are other contributing factors—not exercising or eating well will definitely add to your shoulder problems.

Anatomically speaking the shoulder joint is highly mobile and generally offers a lot of flexibility in various planes of motion. Think of all the different ways that you can move your arm and shoulder compared to your hip which is large, strong and generally stable but limited in flexibility. The flexibility of the shoulders comes at a price—and the price is that shoulder is more easily injured. As you sustain a major injury or a bunch of or "minor" ones you start to loose your flexibility and create the conditions for more serious injuries. This is important to understand because if you are experiencing any chronic symptom in your shoulders it is imperative that you do something about it now—before it gets worse! And it will if you don't pay attention to what is happening in your body.

Remember, pain and discomfort are your bodies messengers. Don't wait. If you are experiencing chronic shoulder symptoms, pick up the phone and call your doctor, chiropractor or physical therapist right this minute! You will be glad you did.

Finally, it is important to know that there is lot you can do right now to help your shoulders and neck. It is easier than you think to become an active participant in your own health. Start by noticing your posture several times through out the day.

- Are you slouching forward or sitting up right with your torso directly over your hips?
- Leaning to one side or another?

- Does your neck crane forward when you are at the computer or is your head neck and spin in one line?
- Are your shoulders close to your ears or relaxed and down away from your ears?

A mantra I like to give my students and clients is: "Lift your collar bones and draw your shoulder blades down your back." Remember these cues and it will go a long way to helping your shoulders and neck.

If you are involved in a job that requires repetitive motions such as computer work, gardening, massage therapy, etc. make sure that you take frequent breaks through out the day. Vary you're the kinds of task you are working on. Repetitive motions for long periods of time put a tremendous amount of stress and strain in your body, leading to injury.

Also, are there any lifestyle issues that are contributing to your shoulder and neck problems? Long periods of driving in your car? Emotional stress? Sports that are aggravating your shoulders? What can be done about these issues? How can they be altered, changed or eliminated so that your shoulders and neck don't take such a beating?

The exercises in this book will help you bring more awareness to your shoulders and neck area, relieve and prevent tightness and pain, release stress overall, and bring needed strength to over stretched body parts.

The relationship between shoulder issues and neck pain

As the old saying goes, the thigh bone is connected to the knee bone, the knee bone connected to the shin bone, and so on and so on. What happens in one part of your body can easily affect another part of your body. This is particularly true for the neck and shoulders for a variety of reasons.

Some of the muscles involved in shoulder movement are located in the neck area. You could say that these muscles are shared by both the neck and shoulders. If you have a problem in these muscles then it is very likely that you will have problems in both your shoulders and your neck.

If you are consistently contracting or overstretching your neck muscles, then your neck will not be supported properly. Disease states, disc issues and strains and sprains in the neck and cervical spine can cause shoulder problems as the body is thrown out of alignment in an effort to compensate for these issues.

The opposite is also true. If you have strained or injured your shoulder or chest muscles then this can effect the postural alignment of your shoulders as well as your neck. Shoulder problems caused by over-use or repetitive activity injuries, lifting and sports injuries can have a profound effect on the neck. When a shoulder is injured, the body will lose its proper postural alignment as it attempts to compensate for the shoulder injury.

Just as there is a relationship between the neck and shoulder muscles there is also a relationship between the cervical vertebra (the part of the spine running through your neck) and the thoracic vertebra (the part of the spine running through your upper back). If the vertebrae in the thoracic spine are not aligned properly, then the cervical spine will most likely be out of alignment.

As you practice the exercises in this book, you will find that some focus more on shoulders and others more on the neck. However you will find that practicing both groups give you the most relief and freedom in your neck and shoulders as one part directly influences the other.

Important considerations for computer users

Did you know that the risk of a muscle-skeletal injury for someone who works on a computer four or more hours per day is nine times greater than it is for a person who spends just one hour per day on the computer? If your job requires a few hours a day or more working on a computer then you are very much at risk for shoulder and neck injuries as well injuries in the back, elbows and wrists.

There are six major reasons why these injuries occur to heavy computer users:

1. Repetitive motions for long periods of time lead to stress and strain on the body
2. Poor posture
3. Work stations set-up improperly; not ergonomically correct
4. Prior injuries / existing weaknesses in the body
5. Little or no regular exercise. (Exercise helps to relieve stress and strengthen the body.)
6. High levels of chronic mental or emotional stress

Any one of the above reasons can in and of itself be the major cause of shoulder or neck issues, and it is also important to realize that injuries are more likely to occur when more than one of these conditions are present. And they often are!

A very common pattern that computer users develop is a rounding of the shoulders and spine and a craning of the neck forward towards the screen. Often this posture is accompanied by raised shoulders. Many people sit like this for hours every day!

This pattern tightens the chest muscles, over stretches the muscles across the shoulder blades, and take the natural curve out of the cervical spine (the part of the spine that runs through your neck area.) Over time, this pattern puts a lot of wear and tear on your body, setting the stage for a variety of shoulder, neck, upper back, arm and wrist injuries.

If this pattern describes your situation then you will benefit greatly from the exercises in this book. All of them will be helpful, but in particular the exercises that focus on stretching the front of the shoulders and the chest while contracting the upper back muscles will be extremely beneficial.

These exercises include the following: Serving tray, Cat balance, One-half dog, Dog on chair, Downward facing dog, Shoulder rolls, Arms front to back, Wall hang, Chest and shoulder opener at wall, Hands up wall, Arms behind interlace fingers and lift, Grab forearm or elbow from behind, Cow's head pose, Locust pose, Bridge pose, Gentle seated twist, Chest opener of the bolster (1 & 2), and Chest opener over blanket.

There are a few more key things you can do help your neck and shoulders if you spend a lot of time on a computer. First, take breaks regularly: a five minute stretch break every hour is ideal. It is also helpful to vary your tasks both on and off the computer. Finally, make sure that you have a good ergonomic setup so you. Consider consulting with an ergonomics specialist or your HR person. They can help you minimize the risk of injury while enhancing productivity. I also have published a good book on the subject entitled: "Office Ergonomics: Preventing Repetitive Motion Injuries and Carpal Tunnel Syndrome" available at www.letsdoyoga.com and www.amazon.com.

Shoulder Anatomy 101

When most people think of their shoulders they think of their deltoids—the muscles on the side of the collar bones that create a "cap" over the upper arm bones or they think of the trapezius muscles which run along the tops of the shoulder from the neck to the upper arm bones. Sometimes people think of their shoulderblades. If you think of your shoulders as any one or all of these landmarks you would be right. But these are just a few of the many, many parts of which the shoulder is made up. As you will see on the next few pages the shoulder is a section of the body that consists of various muscles, bones, joints and connective tissues.

Muscles of the shoulder

The major muscles involved in shoulder movement include the deltoids, trapezius, serratus anterior, infrspinatus, subcapularis, supraspinatus, pectoralis major, pectoralis minor, latissimus dorsi, teres major, teres minor, biceps, triceps, coorcobrachialis, levator scapulae, sternocleidomastoid, and subclavius.

Bones of the shoulder

Scapula (shoulderblades)

Humerus (upper arm bone)

Clavicle (collar bone)

Shoulder joints

Glenohumeral joint: a ball and socket joint located where the upper arm (humerus) and the shoulderblade (scapula) come together.

Acromioclavicular joint: an oval shaped joint where the clavical and acromion meet. The acromion is bony protrusion of the shoulder blades (scapula) that sits just above the top the upper arm bone.

Sternoclavicular: a saddle shaped joint where the clavicles meet at the top of the breast bone (manubrium)

Normal movements of the scapula (shoulder-blade):

The scapula actually floats of over the back of the rib cage aided by muscle, ligaments, and fatty layers and can move the following ways: up, down, away from the centerline of the body, and towards the centerline of the body. The scapula can also move down and in, up while tilting forward into the body, down and out, and towards the front side of the body. The scapula can also move together or independently of each other.

Normal movements of the glenohumeral joint:

Moving the arm forward (flexion)

Moving the arm backward (extension)

Moving the arm out away from the body (abduction)

Moving the arm in towards the centerline of the body (adduction)

Rotating the arm inwards (medial rotation)

Rotating the arm outwards (lateral rotation)

Combination movements involving two or more of the movements just mentioned" such as flexion combined with medial rotation or extension combined with adduction

The movement of the arm overhead is known as the glenohumeral rhythm

Ligaments

Ligaments are connective tissues which join bones to other bones. Shoulder tightness and pain can also be as a result of injured ligaments.

The major ligaments are:

Acromioclavicular and coracoclavicular liagaments; connect the clavicle (collarbone) and acromion which is the high point on top of the scalpula (shoulderblade)

Coracohumeral and glenohumeral ligaments; attach the humerus to the scapula

Coracoacromial ligaments; attach the coracoid process (a bent finger like structure on the front of the scapula) to the acromion

Sternoclavicular ligaments; attaches the sternum(breastbone) and clavicle

Major muscles involved in shoulder movement

Back of body

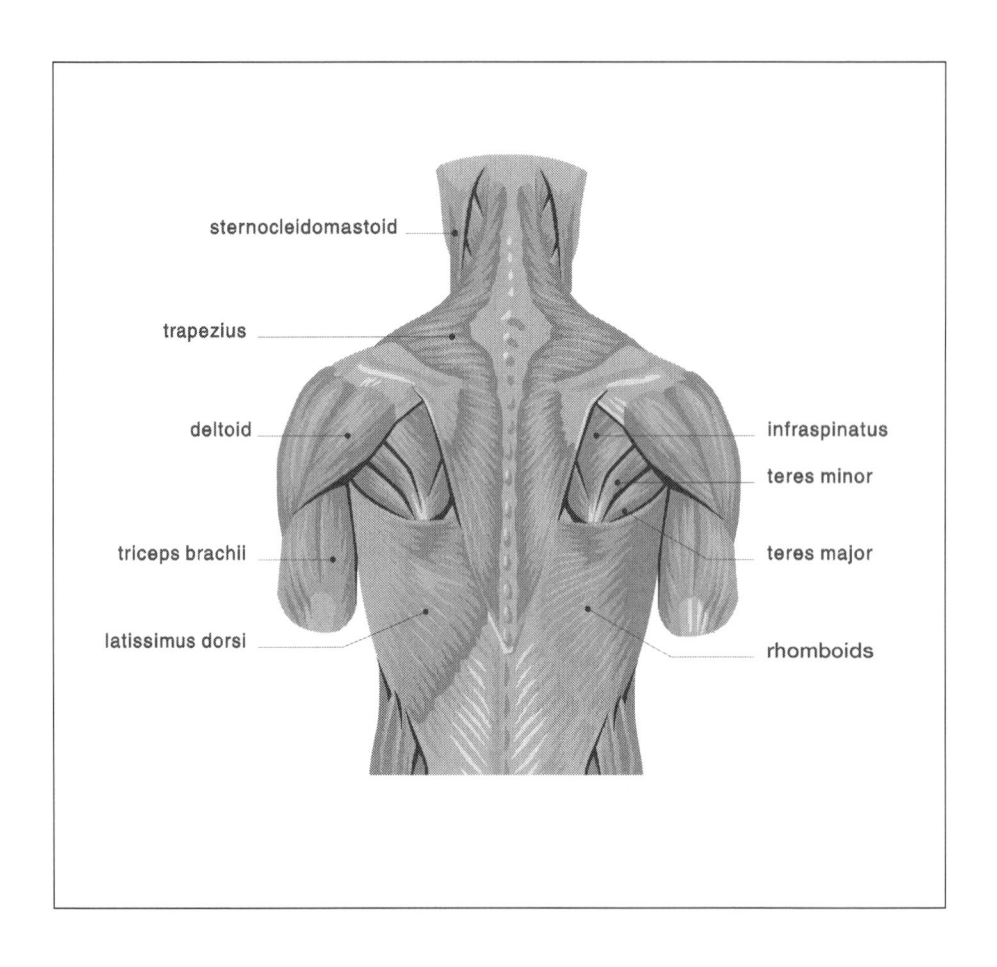

Note: The major muscles involved with movement of the shoulder are shown above and on the next page. Muscles deeper in the body and smaller muscles are not shown.

Front of body

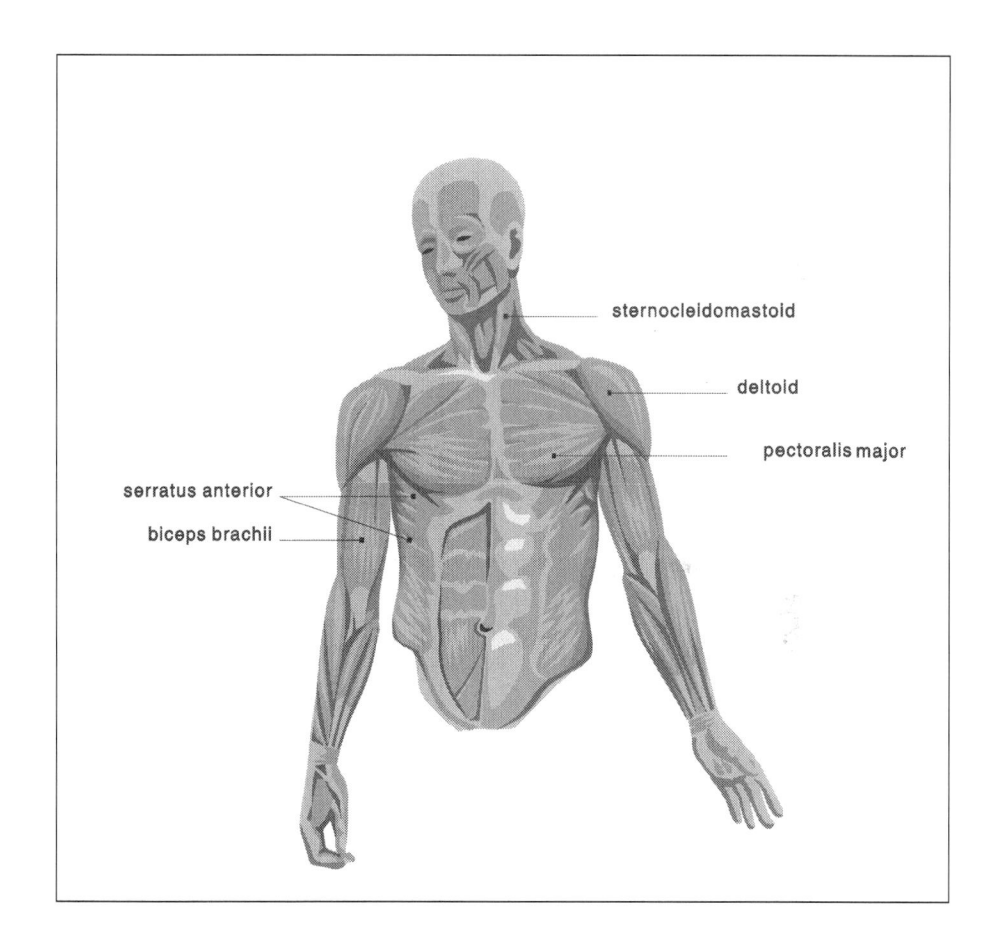

sternocleidomastoid

deltoid

pectoralis major

serratus anterior

biceps brachii

Shoulder Joint

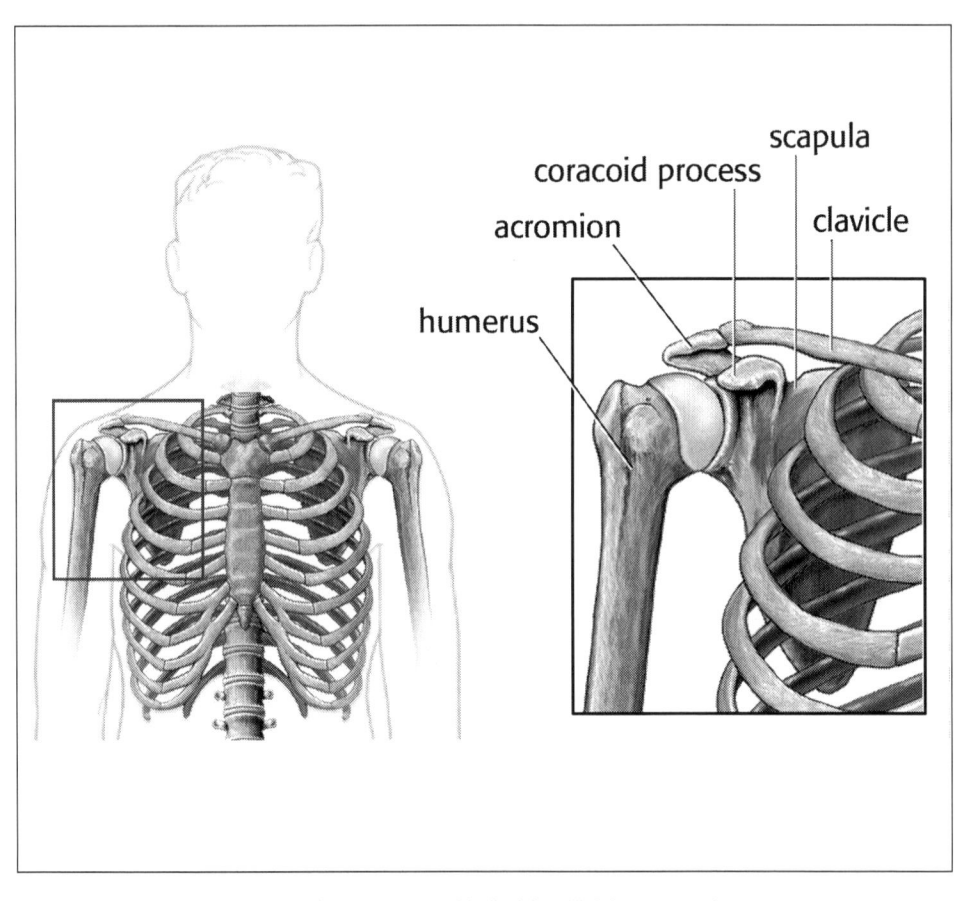

How to Use This Book

The goal of these exercises are to bring your body into balance, provide relief of tight shoulders, improve flexibility, reduce stress and help you feel better in your body.

As you perform the exercises in this booklet you will most likely find that some feel very good to you and that some are challenging. You'll want to feel some sensation in your body but not pain. **Never, never, never** do anything that causes pain, numbness or tingling. These are important messages from your body to either go easier or not do a certain movement at all. Listen to your body! No pain no gain. Right? Wrong! That is how you probably ended up shoulder issues to begin with. Don't ignore your body's signals. Less is definitely more—go easy and be gentle with yourself. The benefits will come—I promise!

Which exercises to do

The exercises are coded by *easy and challenging*. *Easy* exercises are the simplest and safest for most people. *Challenging* exercises require more flexibility as they bring you deeper into your body. Start with a 4 or 5 *easy* exercises and see how this feels in your body. Does it feel good? Was it easy or was it challenging? How did you feel later in the day? Add a few more and work up to 20 to 30 minutes a session over a few weeks. Different exercises will work your shoulders differently—some the front, some the back, some all around, etc. It is good to mix it up with a variety of exercises.

Always start with a few *easy* exercises to warm your body and prepare it for the *challenging* stretches. Be sure to read the instructions for each exercise completely before performing it.

If you have a diagnosed condition in your shoulders such as arthritis, bursitis, frozen shoulder, rotator cuff injury, or disk issues in your neck or upper back, then it is very important to make sure that you perform only the stretches indicated as "easy." As you perform these exercises you want to feel some sensation of stretching, <u>but not pain</u>. If you do feel pain then you need to skip that particular exercise and move on to another, otherwise you are putting yourself at risk for further injury.

If you haven't stretched or exercised your body in some time, you may feel some soreness the next days after you do the exercises. This is ok if it is muscle soreness, but if it is a sharp pain, added discomfort in your joints, numbness or tingling, then these are signs that an exercise was not good for you or you have worked too hard.

If you have an active shoulder or neck issue which you are currently being treated for then it is highly advisable to review the exercises in this book with your physician before practicing them.

How often to practice

Each person has their own unique needs depending on a variety of factors such as what they do for work, stress, pre-existing conditions, genetics, etc. Many people will find relief by practicing these stretches three to five times a week for 20 to 30 minutes each time. If your shoulders are chronically tight then doing a little every day might benefit you. Some people find that 10–15 minutes twice day works best. Those who spend long hours on the computer or perform lots of repetitive movement would do well to take a 5 minute break every hour or so and do a few simple stretches.

Note: An exercise journal has provided for you in the back of this book. Using this journal will help you identify what causes your tight shoulders, track your progress and learn which exercises are most helpful.

A common pattern

A common pattern among many people who have tight shoulders is for the chest to collapse—the muscles in the front of the chest tighten as the shoulders move forward and up. If this describes the condition of your shoulders be sure to find the exercises that open your chest—stretch your pectoral muscles. You will find the exercises in section entitled "Additional Ideas of Interest" a great relief!

How Breathing Affects Your Shoulders & Neck

There is a direct connection between your breath and your shoulders and neck, not to mention your energy and the way your feel. When your breath is deep you will find that your chest and shoulders are open and your head naturally lifts helping to bring your neck into proper alignment. This alignment is consistent with good energy. The opposite is also true; when your chest is collapsed and your shoulders forward then your breathing with be restricted as well. This position is often associated with depression or sadness. Try it for yourself right now. First roll your shoulders forward, letting your chest collapse and your head droop. How is your breath? How do feel energetically? Now do the opposite. Lift and broaden your chest, elongate your spine and take a few deep breaths. How is your breath now? Easier? Deeper? How is your energy? How do your shoulders feel? Remember your breath, your posture/shoulders and the state of your mind are intimately linked. One effects the other.

As you enhance your ability to breath you will enjoy a number of important benefits: You will improve your oxygen intake which will result in more energy which in-turn will activate the mechanism that brings balance to your mind and emotions thereby reducing the effect of stress. You will also be improving your posture and in the process open your chest and shoulders and help the alignment of your neck and head. By becoming more aware of your breath you will be come more aware of your posture and what is happening your shoulders.

Here's how to breathe

Sit in a comfortable, bringing your head, neck and spine into one line. Place your hands on your chest and breath in and out through your nose, feeling your chest expand. Do this three times. This is a chest breath, rather shallow and is the breath that is associated with tension and anxiety—especially when it is quick and your mouth open.

Now place your hands on your belly. Inhale through your nostrils and as you do this let your belly expand filling the entire abdominal area with your breath. Exhale through your nose and press in slightly with your hands. Repeat this three times. This is the diaphragmatic breath that begins to activate your parasympathetic nervous system (relaxation response). Think of a baby resting or sleeping—how easy and naturally the belly moves in and out.

Next, place your left palm on your chest and your right palm on your belly. As you inhale through your nose let your belly expand and then bring your breath up into your chest, feeling your ribs expand. Exhale through your nose slowly, releasing your breath first from your chest and then your stomach. Repeat three more times. Now close your eyes, rest your hands on your lap and repeat this breath five times. Notice how you feel after you breath this way. How is your energy—relaxed and focused? How about the position of your shoulders?

Note: If you find this breath is difficult for you or you feel it makes you feel anxious then just focus on the belly breath portion. Make you exhalations a little slower than your inhalations. Remember to lift and broaden through your chest though.

On occasion you may experience a feeling of tiredness after performing the complete breath. This is because your anxiety level has dropped and the underlying tiredness is allowed to surface. Keep breathing and in time you will feel better.

Schedule many breathing breaks during the day to check-in with your shoulders and to take a 5 to 10 deep breaths. You feel better and so will your shoulders! Try it and see for yourself.

Exercises

Side stretch on back
Easy

Lie on your back with your legs extended. Walk your legs a little to the left until you feel a stretch in the right side of your torso. Take your right arm up overheard behind you and stretch through your right arm and out through your finger tips. Take five deep breaths and release. Do the other side.

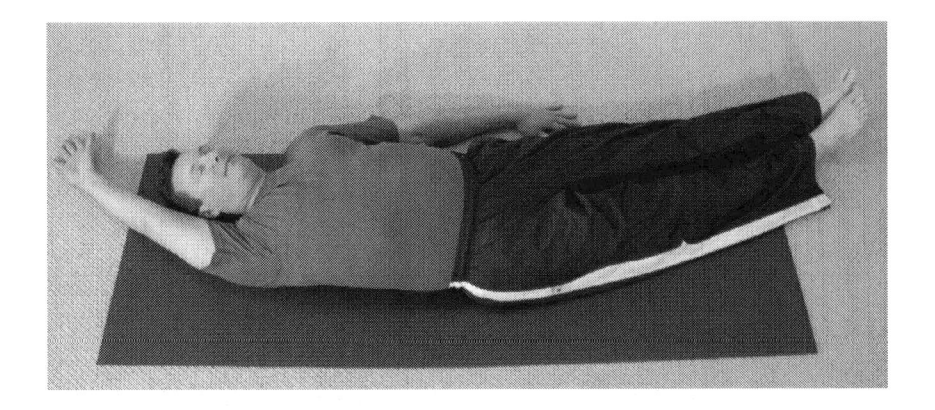

Serving tray

Easy

Lie on your back with legs extended. Place a book or yoga block in the palm of your right hand as if your were holding a serving tray. Now take the book over head behind you, extending through your right arm. If you are feeling pain or too much stretch, try it without a book or use a foam yoga block instead. Take five deep breaths and do the other side.

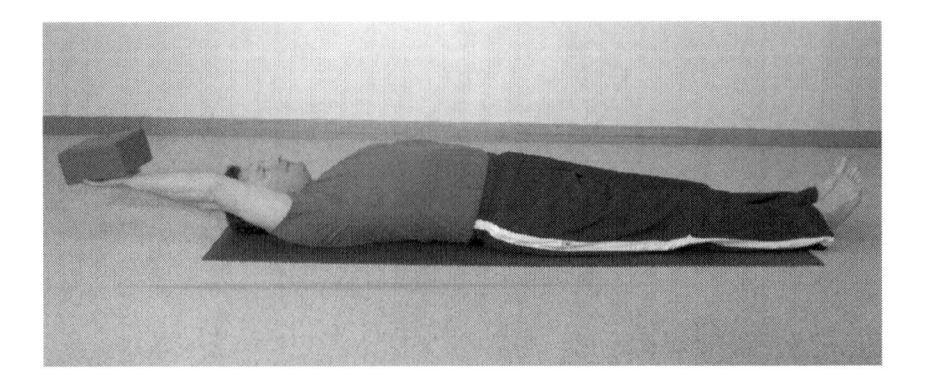

Cat tuck and dog tilt
Easy

As you exhale, bring your head and hips towards each other arching like a cat. Lift your belly button up towards your spine. This is cat tuck. Release, inhale, and turn your tail bone up towards the sky, rotating your hips over the tops of your thighs. At the same time lift your head and chest. This is dog tilt. Go back and forth from cat tuck to dog tilt several times. Go slowly and use your breath.

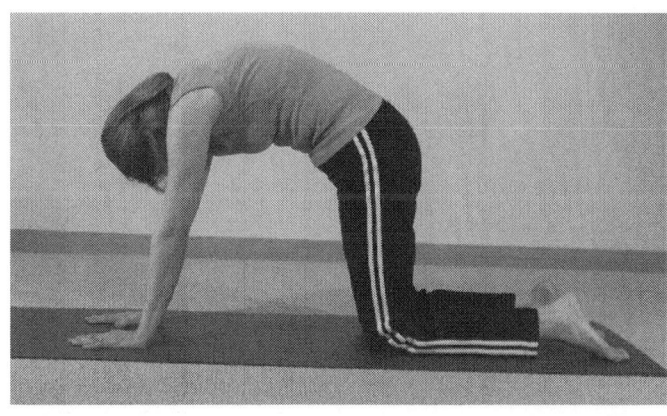

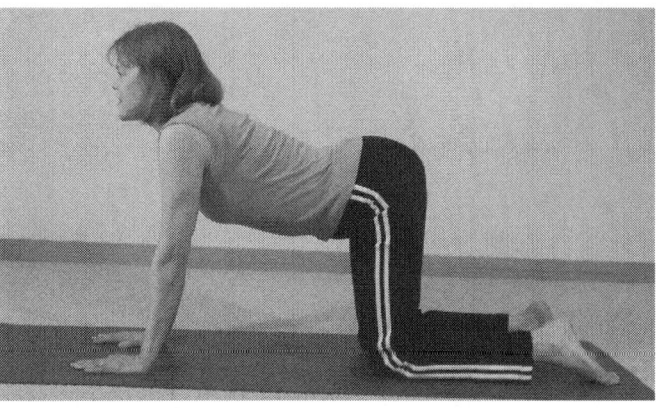

Cat balance
Easy

Come onto all fours with your arms right under your shoulders and your knees right under your hips. Extend your right leg back directly behind you and then extend your left arm straight out in front. Hold for five breaths and then repeat on the other side. As a variation go from side to side holding for just one breath.

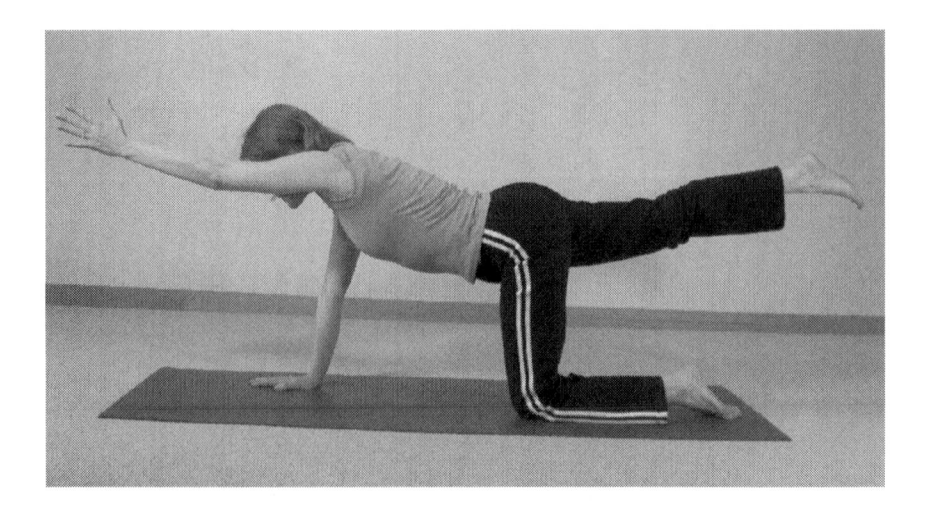

Child

Easy

Come onto all fours with your arms under your shoulders and knees right under your hips. As you exhale bring your hips towards your calves and chest towards your thighs. Bring your hands along side of your shins, palms facing up. Take five to ten breaths. If your head does not comfortably touch the floor, place a folded blanket under your head. As a variation you can extend your arms in front of you. This stretches the shoulders in a different way than having your arms along side of your shins and is a good preparation for the next exercise.

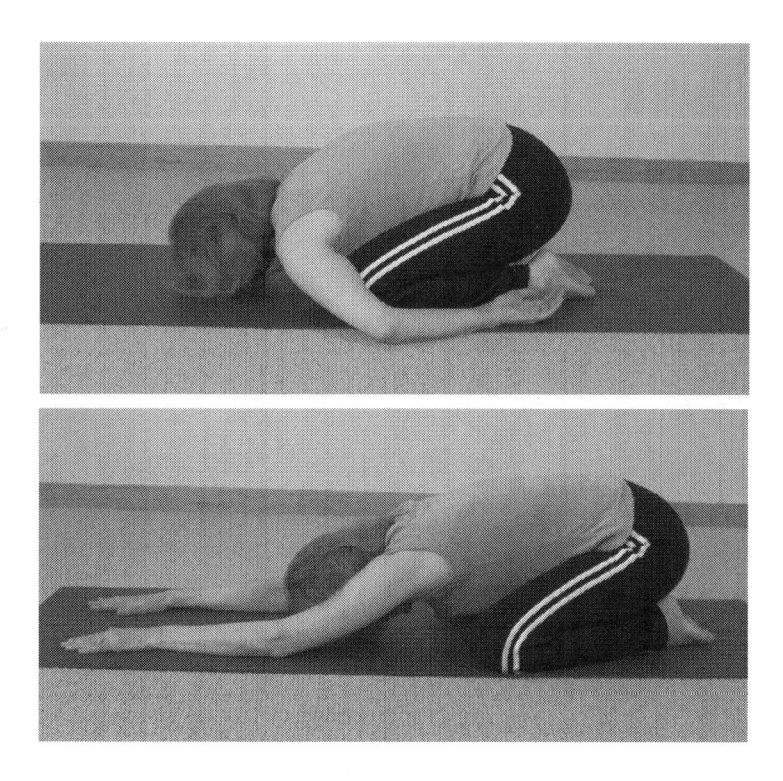

Child–extended to the side

Easy

As you exhale bring your hips towards your calves and chest towards your thighs. Extend your arms out in front of you. If you head does not comfortably touch the floor, place a blanket under your head. Keeping your head between your arms walk your arms to the right. You should feel a good stretch through the left side of your torso—breath into this stretch. For more intensity press the left shoulder down slightly. Take five to eight breaths, release, and do the other side.

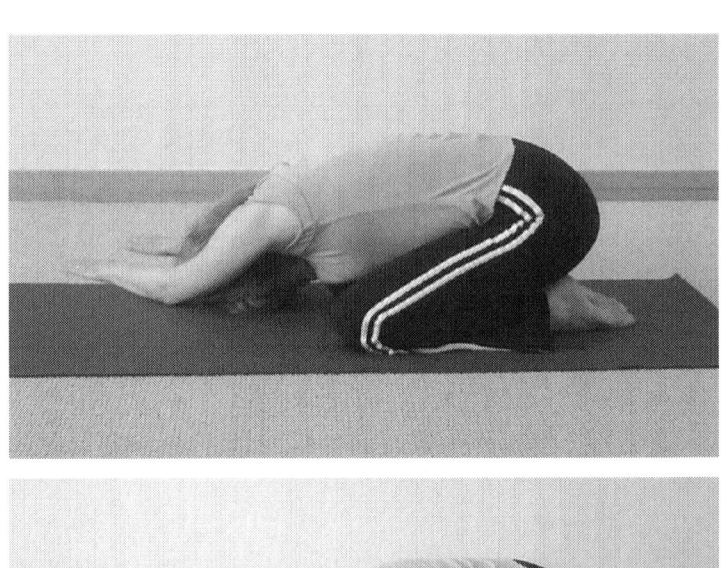

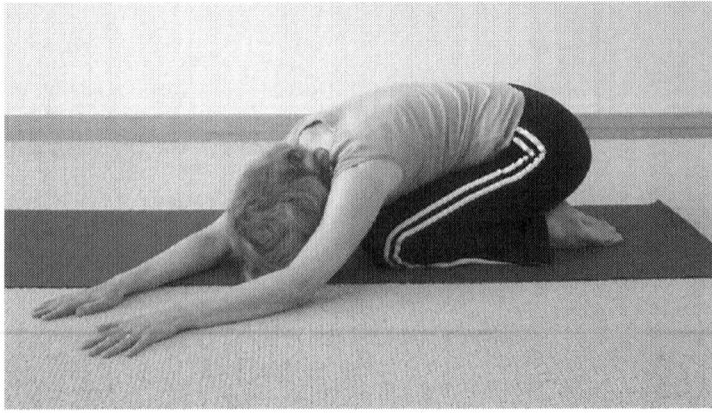

One-half dog

Easy

Come onto all fours with your arm under your shoulders knees right under your hips. Keeping your hips over your knees, slowly walk your hands forward until your arms are fully extended.

If you forehead does not comfortably touch the floor, lift your head so that you ears are inline with your arms. You may also put a blanket under your head. Do not put a lot of force on your shoulders. Take five to ten breaths.

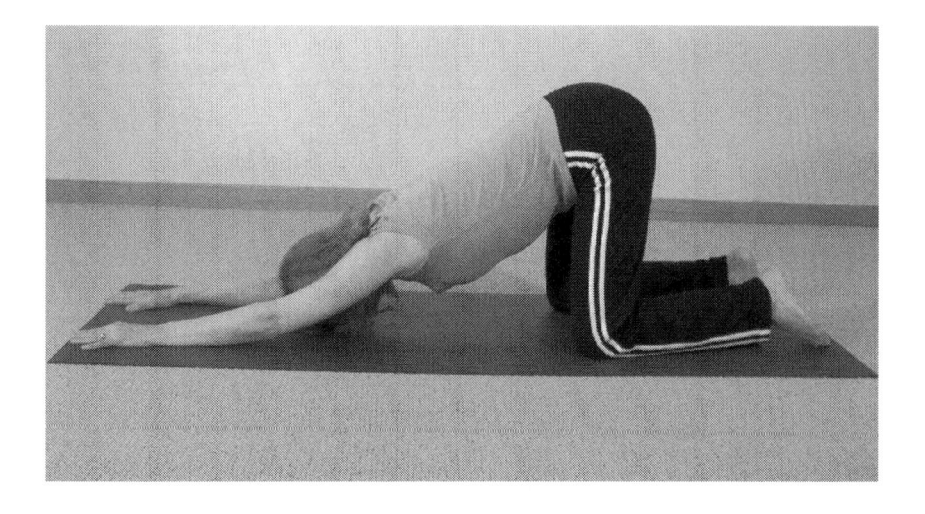

Downward facing dog
Challenging

Come onto all fours with your arm under your shoulders knees right under your hips. Walk your hands forward a few inches so your arms are in front of your shoulders. Make sure your middle finger is pointing straight ahead and spread your fingers wide. Curl you toes onto the floor. As you exhale press into your hands and lift your hips up towards the ceiling. Stay on your toes for a moment. Press your hands into the floor and lift your hips higher. Now, from the height of your hips press your heels towards the floor. Press your hands into the floor again, lengthen through your arms, lengthen through the sides of your chest and waist. Press your thighbones towards your hamstrings and stretch down into your heels. Take five to ten breaths and come down into child position to rest. If this posture hurts your shoulders or if you don't have the strength for it practice one-half dog instead on a chair.

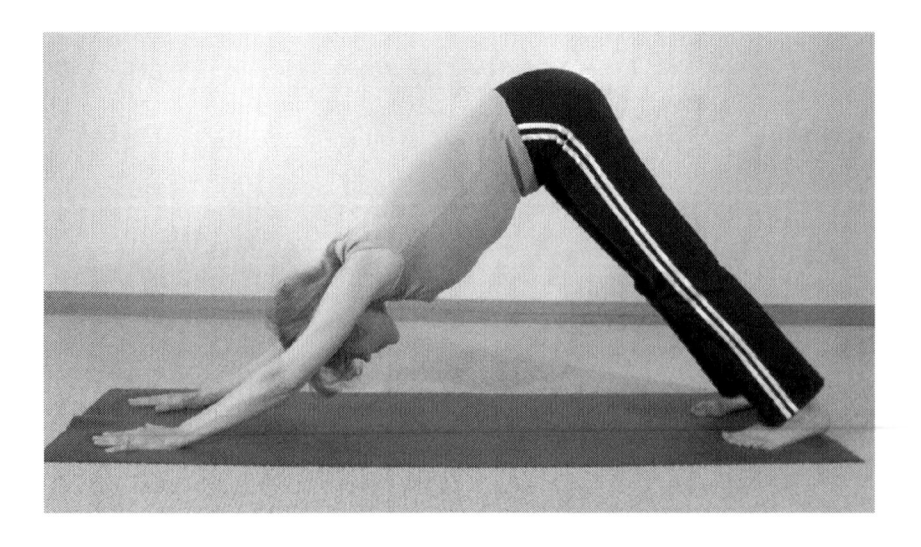

Dog on chair
Easy

Place a chair against a wall or on a yoga mat as shown in photo. Standing in front of the chair, place your palms on the chair seat and walk your feet back until they are a little behind your hips. Make sure your arms are in-line with your shoulders and your feet are hips width apart. Press down evenly on your palms and lengthen through you arms and the sides of your torso. Take your hips back more. Take five to ten breaths. Walk your feet towards the chair to come out of the pose.

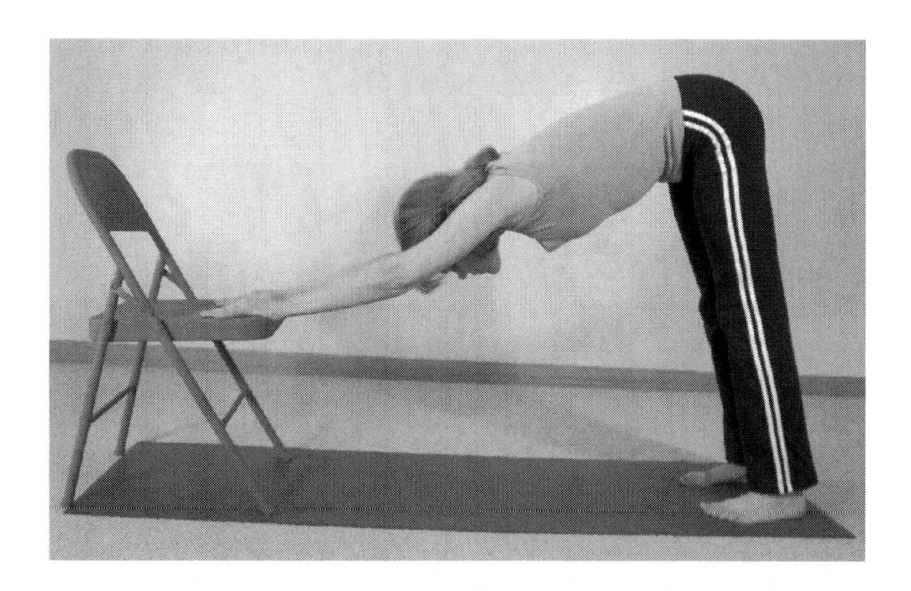

Shoulder rolls

Easy

Stand with your legs right under your hips and feet pointing straight ahead. Lift up through your spine and broaden through your chest. S-l-o-w-l-y roll your shoulders forward three to five times and then roll them backwards three to five times.

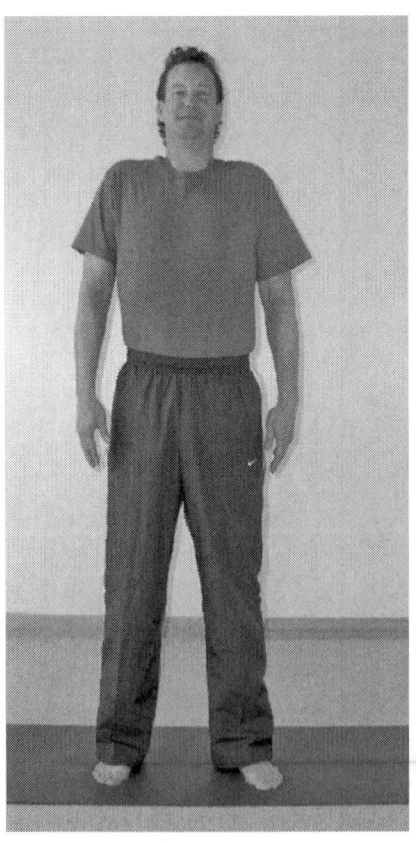

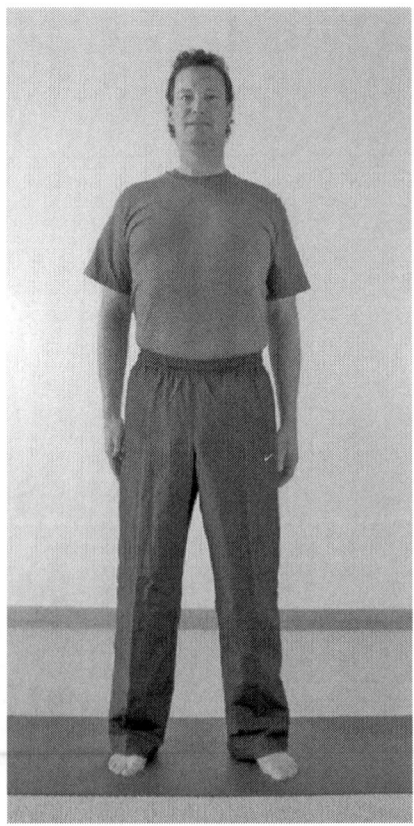

Shoulder shrugs
Easy

Stand with your legs right under your hips and feet pointing straight ahead. Lift up through your spine and broaden through your chest. As you inhale bring your shoulders up towards your ears, hold for a second or two and then with a big exhale (through your mouth) release your shoulders away from your ears. Repeat three to five times.

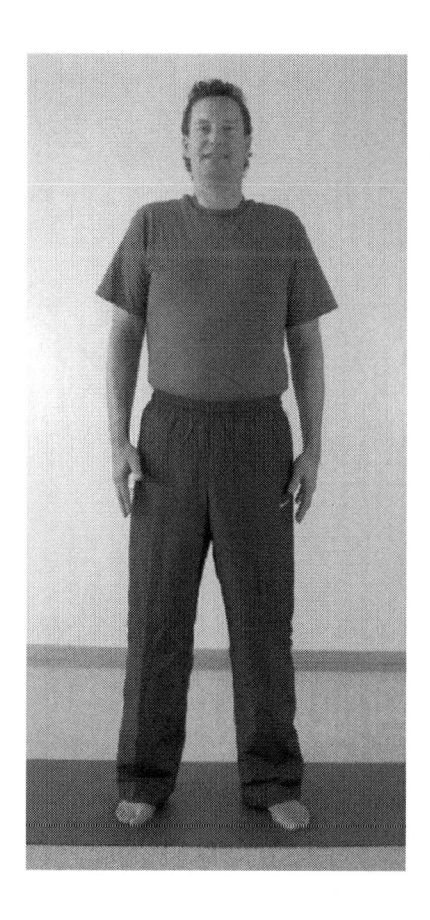

Arm extended to side with hand on head

Easy

Stand with your legs right under your hips and feet pointing straight ahead. Lift up through your spine and broaden through your chest. Extend your left arm to the side at shoulder height. Place your right hand on your left ear and very gently bring your right ear towards your right shoulder.

Reach through your left arm. Take five deep breaths and repeat on the other side.

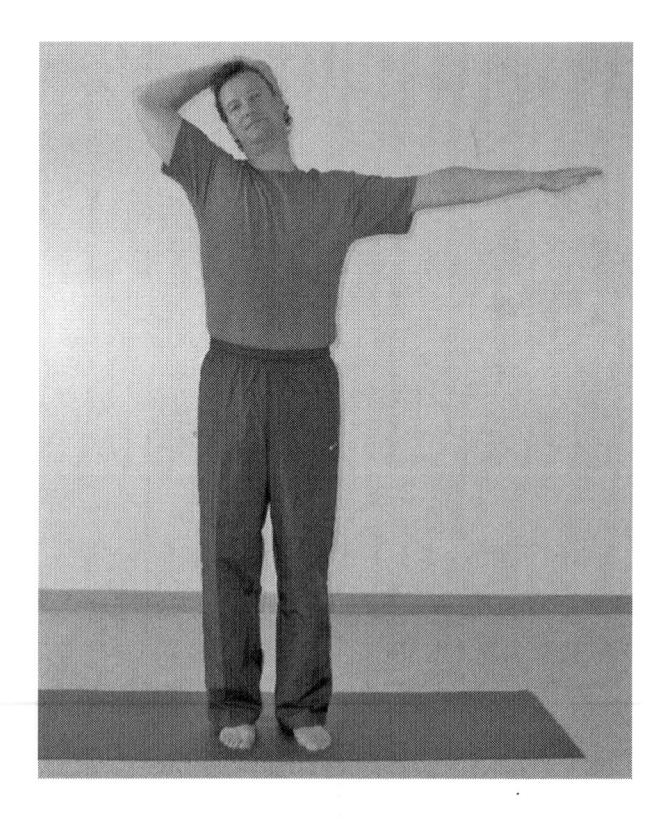

Pat on the back
Easy

Stand with your legs right under your hips and feet pointing straight ahead. Lift up through your spine and broaden through your chest. Bring your right hand across the top of your left shoulder. Let your hand rest on your torso—it may be on the top of your shoulder or on the shoulderblade side. Place your left hand on your right elbow and push gently towards your torso. Hold for five to eight breaths. This is a great stretch for the back of the shoulderblade.

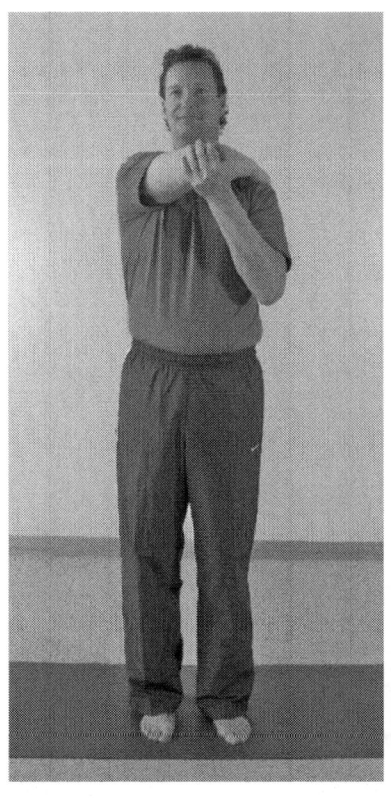

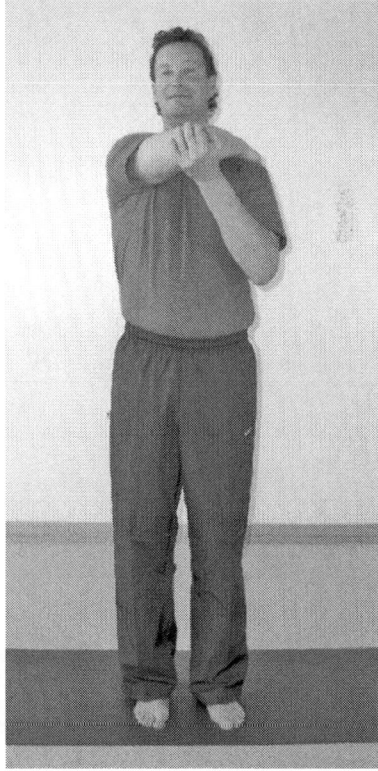

Arm swings
Easy

Stand with your legs right under your hips and feet pointing straight ahead. Lift up through your spine and broaden through your chest. Extend your arms out in front of you at the height of your mid-chest. Swing your left arm over your right as you move your left arm to the right. At the same time swing your right under your left. Keep your arms loose as you swing them. Keep moving the arms back and forth, changing which arm is on top. Repeat several times

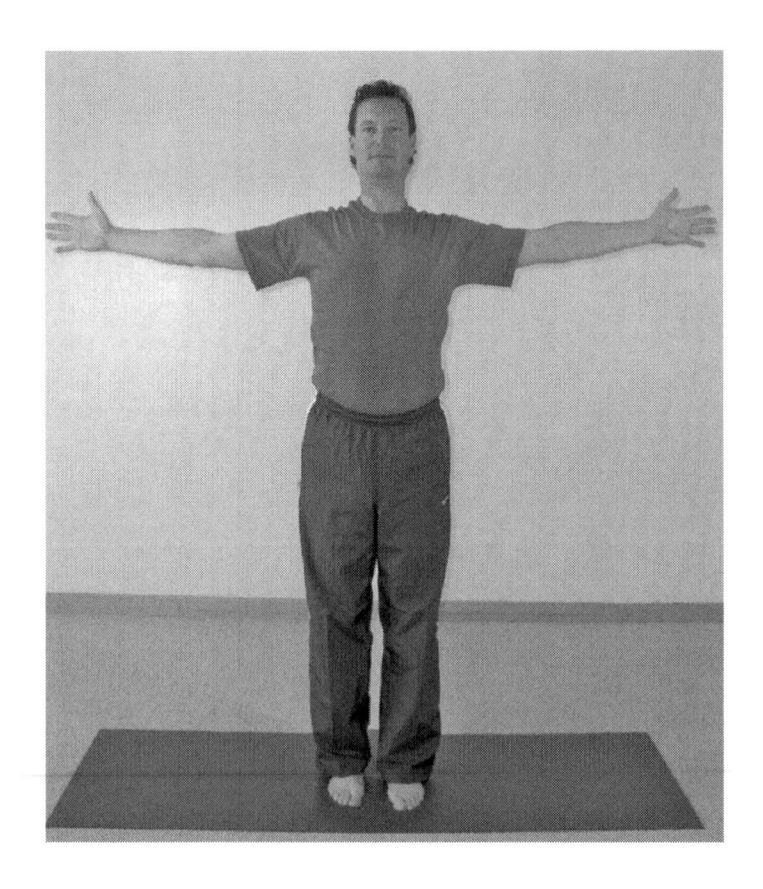

Tight Shoulder Relief Tip

Take a break! If you shoulders are chronically tight due to a job that requires a lot of repetitive motions such as those needed by a heavy computer user, dental hygienist or hair stylist be sure to give yourself a break every hour or so for 5 minutes. Do a little stretching or go for a walk. Remember to take a break! Your shoulders will thank you and you'll have better mental energy too!

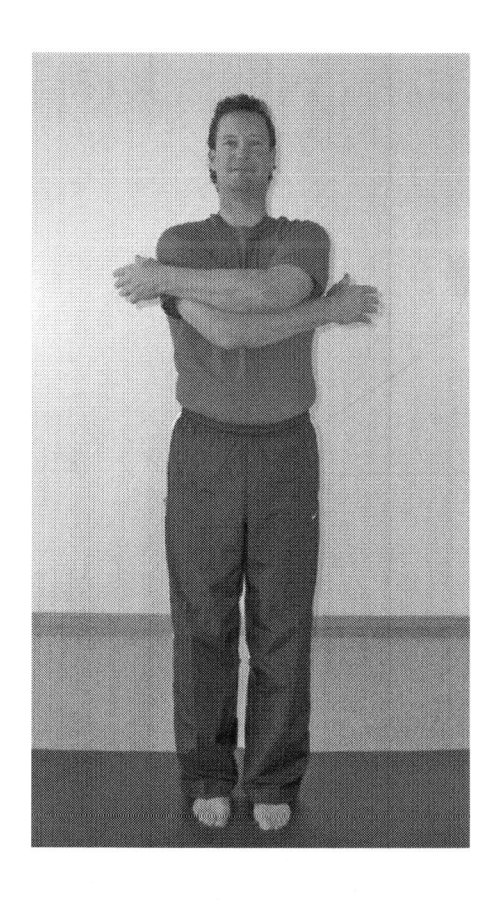

Arms up and down
Easy

Stand with your legs right under your hips and feet pointing straight ahead. Lift up through your spine and broaden through your chest. With your arms at your sides, turn your palms out away from your body. As you inhale, slowly lift your arms up overhead until the palms touch, turn your palms out and then exhale and lower your arms, bringing your hands back to your sides. Repeat five times.

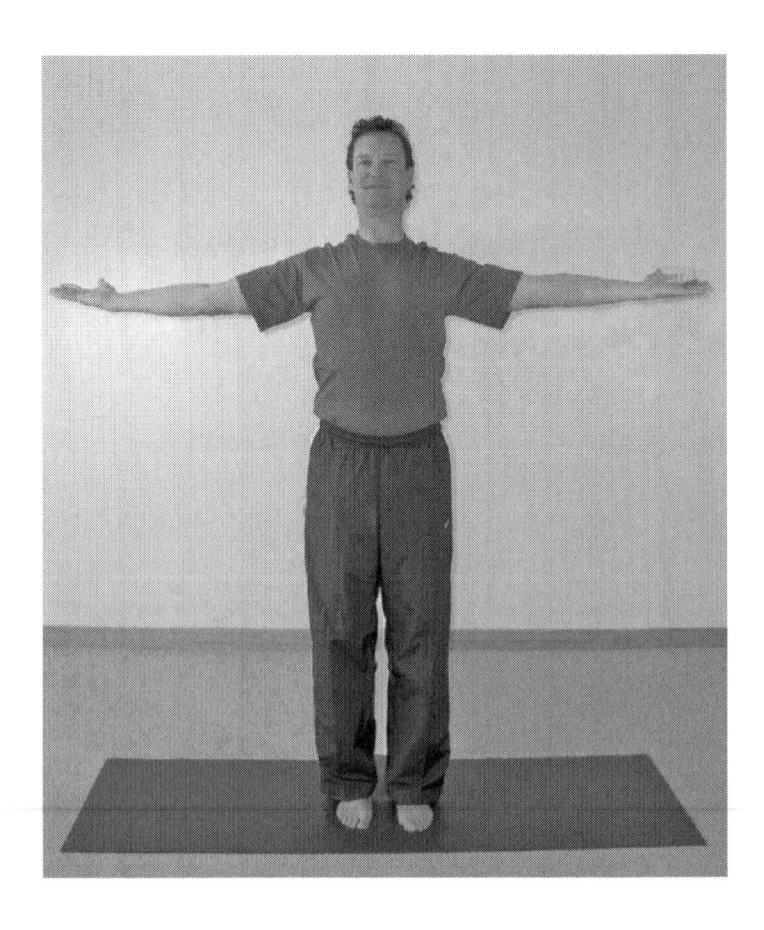

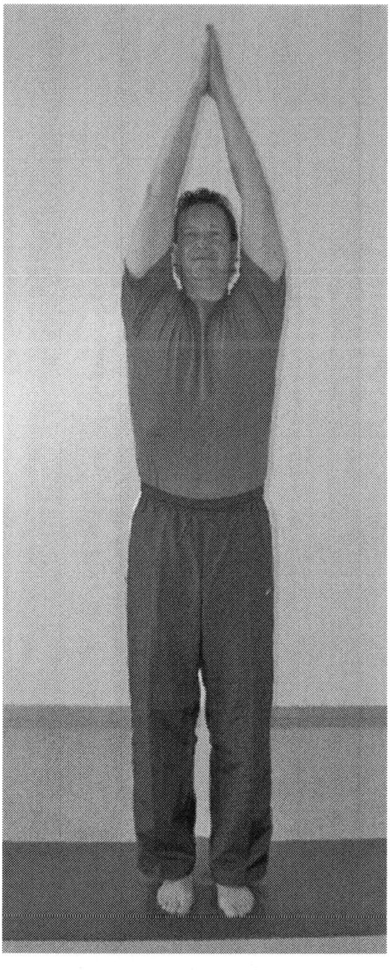

Arms front to back

Easy

Stand with your legs right under your hips and feet pointing straight ahead. Lift up through your spine and broaden through your chest. With your arms at your sides turn the palms forward.

As you inhale take your arms back behind you, lifting and open your chest. As you exhale bring them forward so the palms touch in front of you. Now take your arms a little higher and repeat the motion. Take the arms a total of four steps higher until they are a little above your shoulders and then start to work your way down the way you came up. Focus on making the forward and backward arm motions smooth and coordinate these movements with your breath—inhaling as you take your arms back and exhaling as you take them forward.

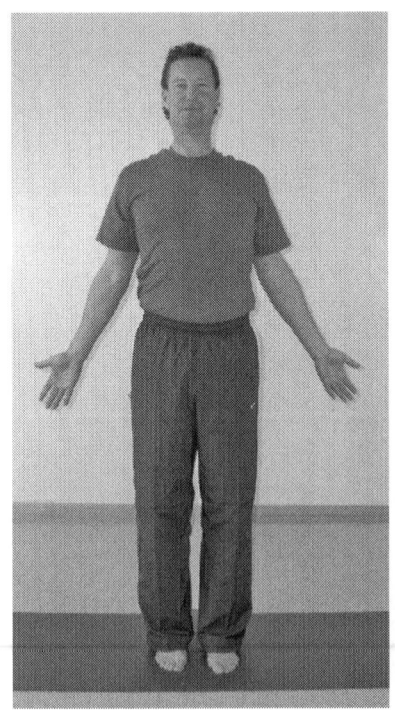

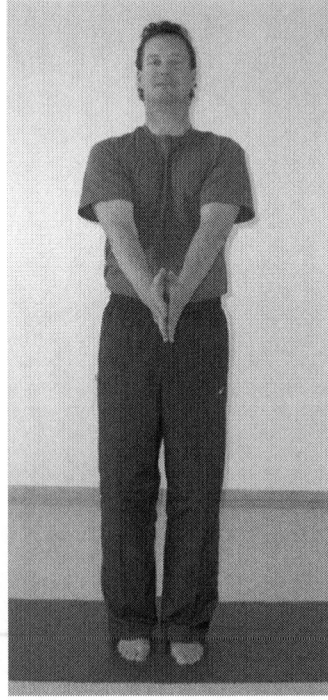

Tight Shoulder Relief Tip

Become a detective! Identify what is contributing to your tight shoulders. Is it too much time working on a computer? Emotional stress? Driving a car too much? Bad posture? Old injury? What specifically is contributing to your shoulder discomfort? Once you have identified the cause, ask yourself what can be changed to reduce or eliminate this stressor.

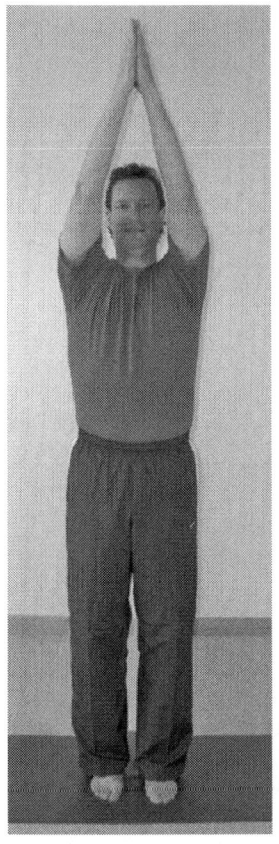

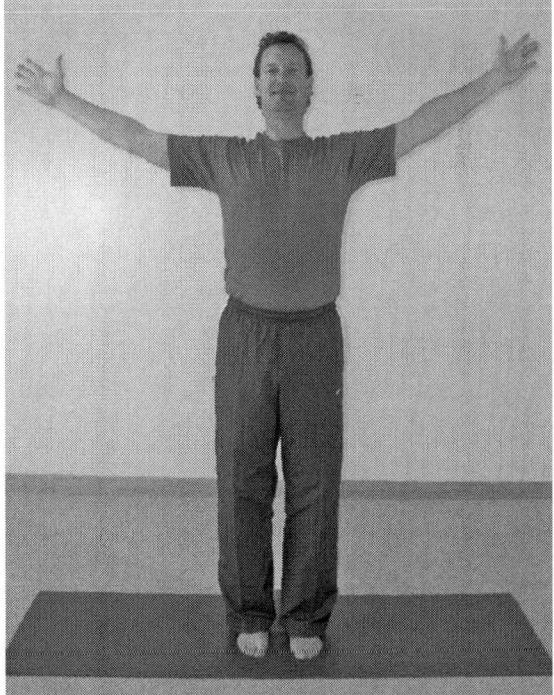

Mountain

Easy

Stand with your legs right under your hips and feet pointing straight ahead. Pull up on your thighs (quadriceps). Be sure not to hyperextend your knees. Lift up through your spine. Lift the sides of your chest. Broaden through your top chest releasing the outside of your shoulders down towards your hips. Reach out through the crown of your head. As you inhale take your arms out the sides at shoulder height with the palms up. Pause here and from the center of you chest stretch into your finger tips. Take a few breaths. On your next inhale lift your arms straight up towards the ceiling with palms facing each other. Lift your arms strongly to lift the sides of your chest and waist. Hold for a few breaths and release.

Note: if for some reason it feels uncomfortable to lift your arms from the sides try taking them in front of you and then overhead.

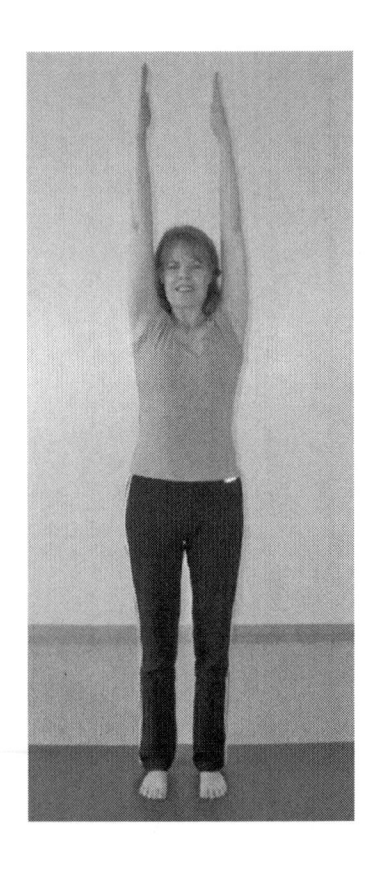

Mountain with side stretch
Easy

Follow directions on the previous page for Mountain. With arms extended overhead turn your left palm out (away from your body). Grab your left forearm with your right hand and pull up gently. As you exhale press into your left hip taking your left arm over head. Press into your left foot and stretch all the way into your left hand. Keep your right shoulder and left shoulder in line with each other. Also keep your chin off your chess so that your head neck and spine are in one line. Hold for five breaths and then inhale to come up. Repeat on the other side.

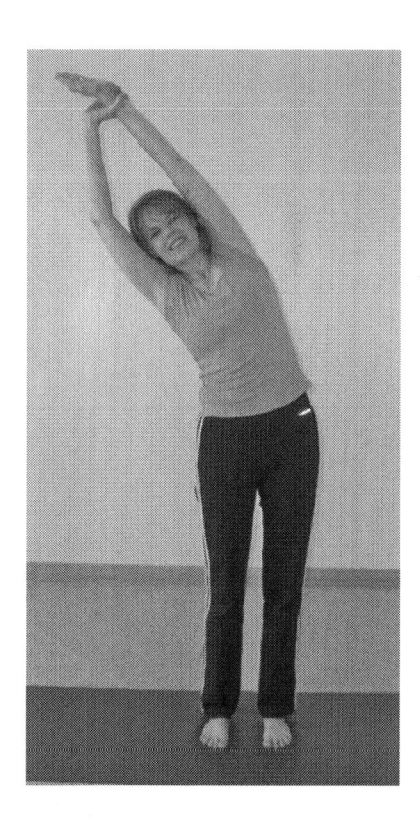

Wall hang

Easy

Stand a few inches away from a wall (facing the wall). Put your finger tips on the wall even with your mid chest area. Keeping your finger on the wall walk your feet back until your torso is more or less parallel to the ground. Your legs should be right under your hips (front to back) and hip width apart. Lengthen through your arms and stretch into your hips. Ideally you will want to end up with your arms and sides of your shoulders in one line. Take five to ten slow breaths. If you have tight shoulders you most likely will need to take your hands a few inches higher up the wall to be in the proper position. It may be hard to determine this at first on your own so consider having someone else look at your posture in this exercise.

Note: If it hurts your hands to use your fingertips come onto your palms instead. Be sure not to sink into your shoulders; instead lengthen through them.

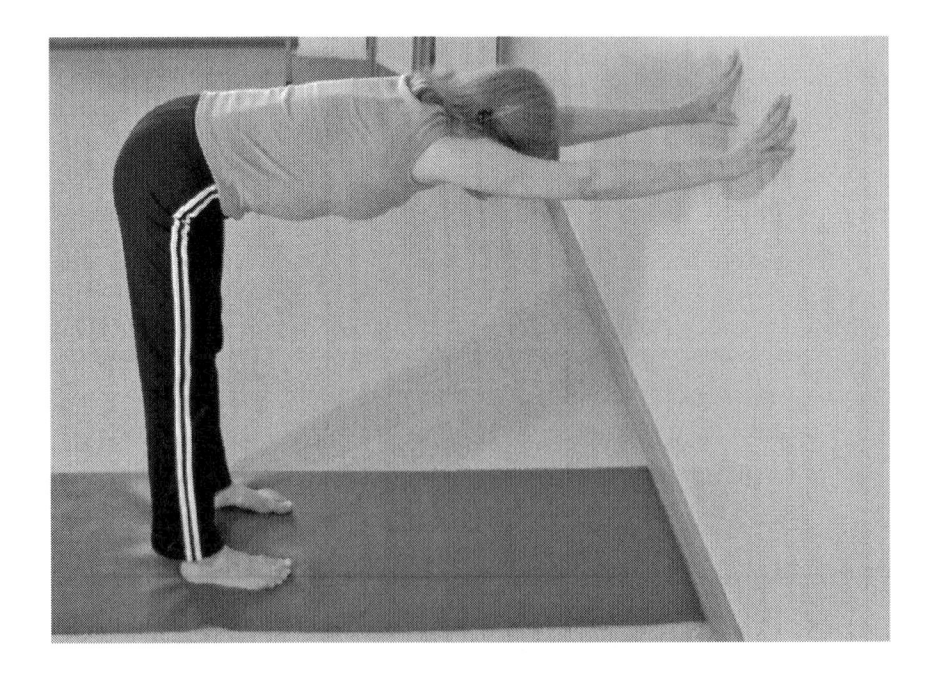

Tight Shoulder Relief Tip

Get a quickie! A quick 5–10 minute chair massage is a great way to relieve tight shoulders and neck muscles. Many companies have a massage therapist come to their office regularly for this very purpose. If your company doesn't maybe a group of employees and can share the fee of having a massage therapist visit during lunch or a scheduled break. Chair massage can also often be found at health food stores such as Whole Foods for a very reasonable fee.

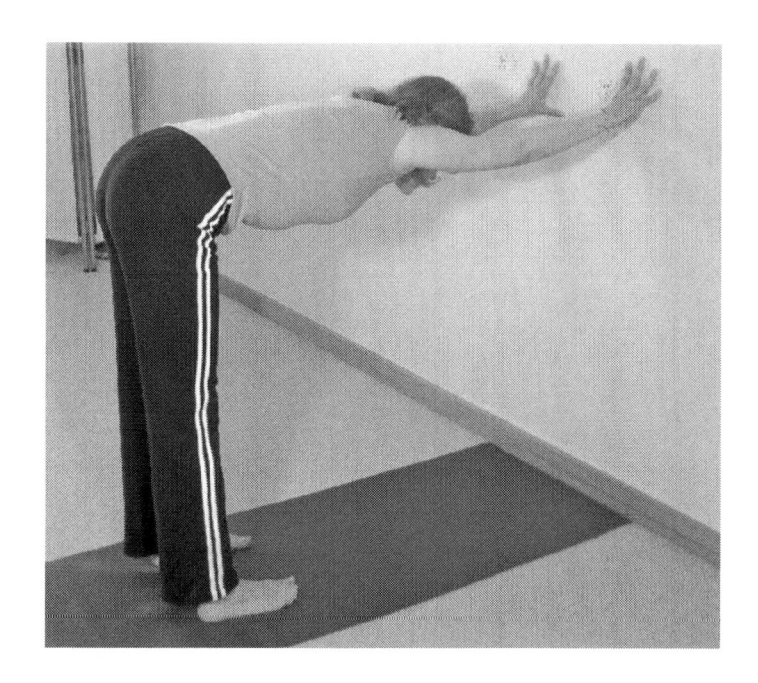

Wall hang—turn fingers in/out
Challenging

Follow the directions for Wall hang. Instead having your fingertips on the wall place your palms on the wall with your fingertips of one hand facing the fingertips of the other. It is important to make sure your wrist are in line with your shoulders. Take five slow breaths and turn your fingers the other way—so that they are facing out, away from each other. Again, make sure your wrists are in line with your shoulders. Take five breath and release.

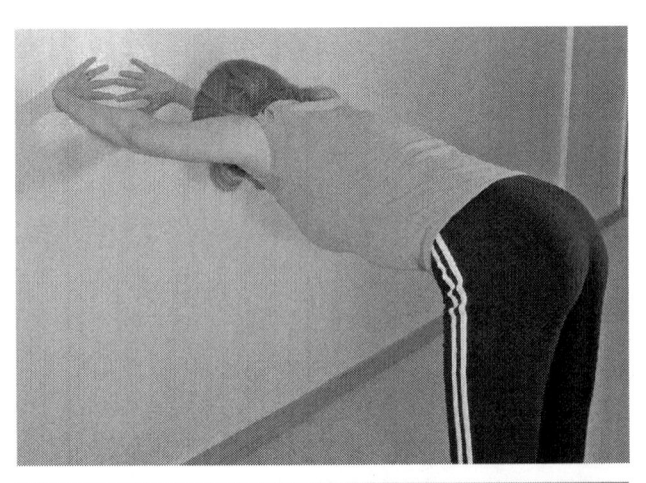

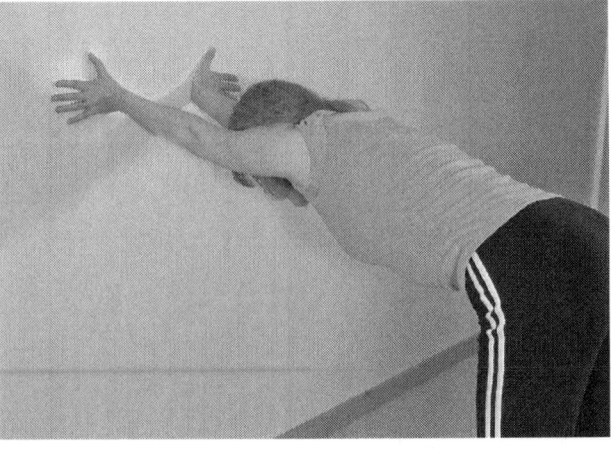

Chest and shoulder opener at wall
Challenging

Stand with the right side of your body facing a wall. Be arms length from the wall. Bring your finger tips onto the wall at shoulder height and turn your hand clockwise approximately five minutes on a clock face. Slowly walk your feet to the left until you feel a good stretch in your shoulder, chest or arm. Keep you hips and torso over your hips as you turn. If you want more stretch walk your feet a little more to the left. For less stretch walk your feet to the right. Take five to eight slow deep breaths and release. Repeat on the other side. As a variation you can bring your left hand to the outside of your right pectoral muscle (chest muscle) and gently pull away from your arm.

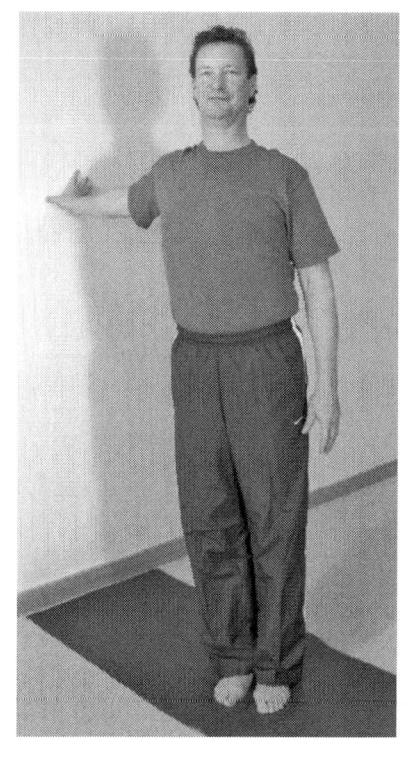

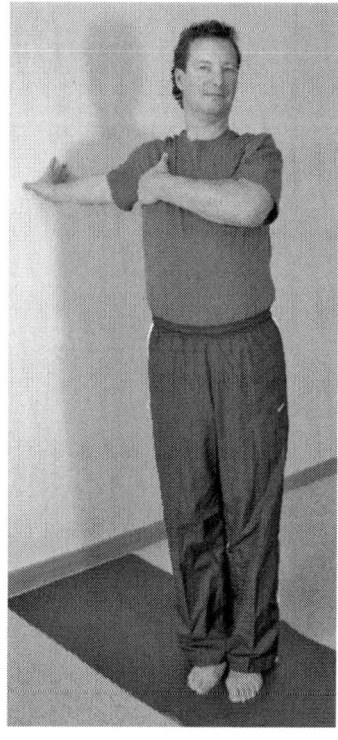

Arm up wall
Easy

Stand with the right side of your torso facing the wall. Bring the right side of your rib cage up against the wall. Extend your right arm up overhead placing the palm of your right hand on the wall. If this hurts your shoulder don't do this exercise. Now lift both heels about two inches off the ground. Imagine that your right hand is glued to the wall and very s-l-o-w-l-y lower your right hip away from your right hand so that the whole right side of your upper body is stretching. When the right heel touches the floor bring the left heel to the floor. Release and do the other side.

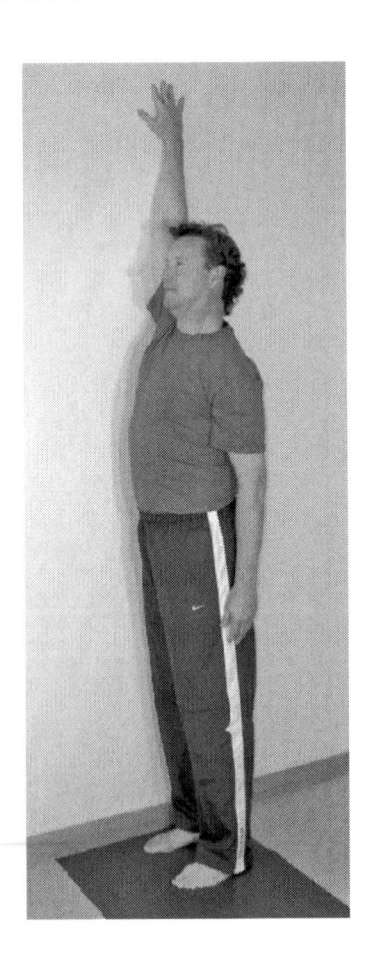

Hands up the wall
Easy

Stand about six inches away from a wall. Extend your arms overhead and place your palms on the wall. Lower your forehead to the wall. Do not force your forehead to the wall. It is OK if it doesn't touch. Keeping your hands and forehead on the wall start to move your feet back until you feel a good stretch in your shoulders, arms or chest.

If you feel discomfort in your neck or shoulders lift your forehead off the wall. Make sure you are not overarching your lower back. For less stretch walk your feet in towards the wall for more stretch walk your feet back. Take five to ten deep breaths and release.

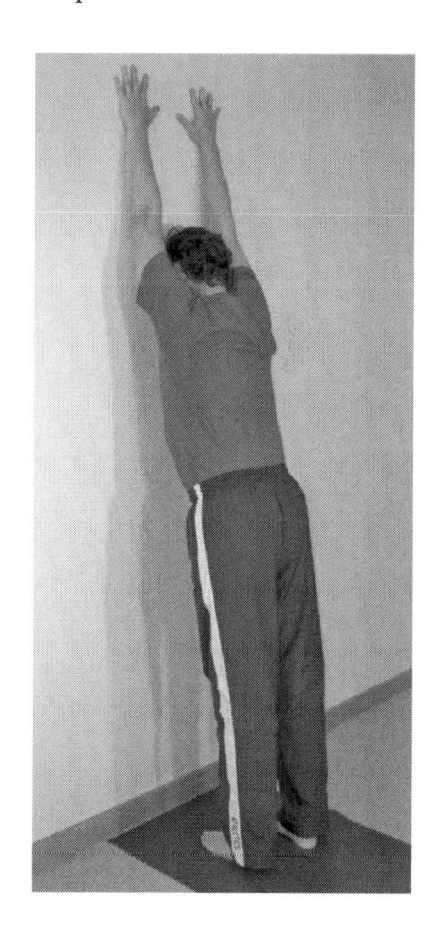

Arm circles at wall
Easy

Stand with the right side of your body facing a wall. Be about four to six inches from the wall. Take you right arm straight up and reach through your finger tips. Slowly begin to make a complete circle in a clockwise direction. Repeat three to four times. And then make circles in the counter clockwise position. Release and do the other side.

Note: If it is difficult to complete the circle or if you feel pain then step a few inches further from the wall and try again.

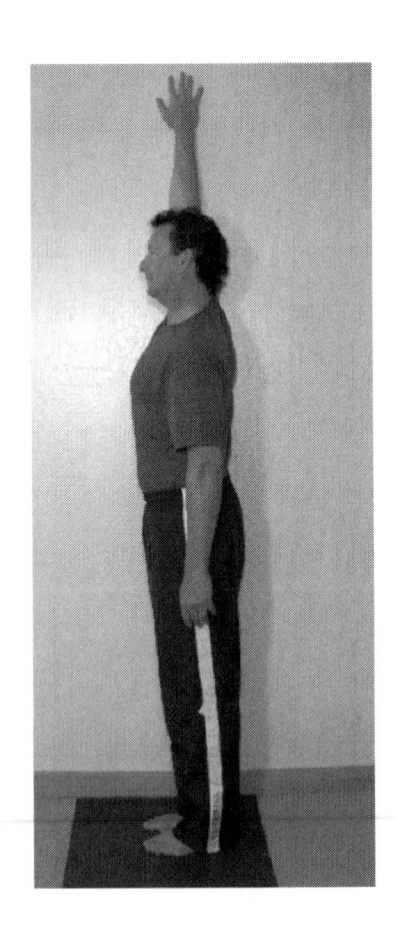

Tight Shoulder Relief Tip

Heat it up! A great way to relieve tight shoulders and reduce pain is with heat. Consider using a hot pack that you can just through in a microwave and then put on your shoulders. Or go low tech and soak a towel in hot water, squeeze the water out and put it on your shoulders. A hot shower, bath, sauna or steam are also very effective options for soothing your shoulders and relieving stress.

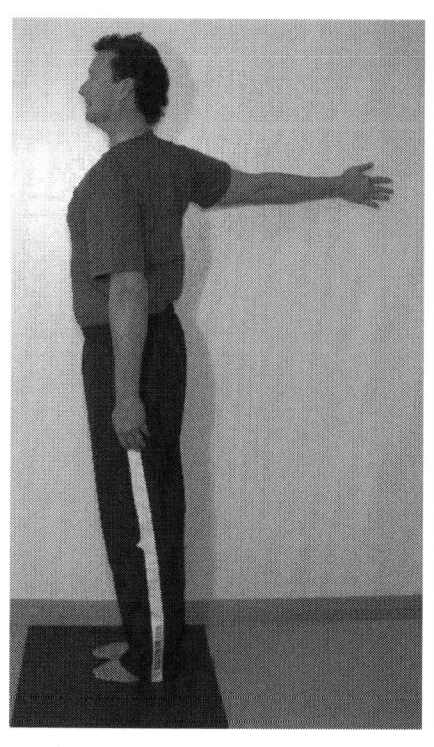

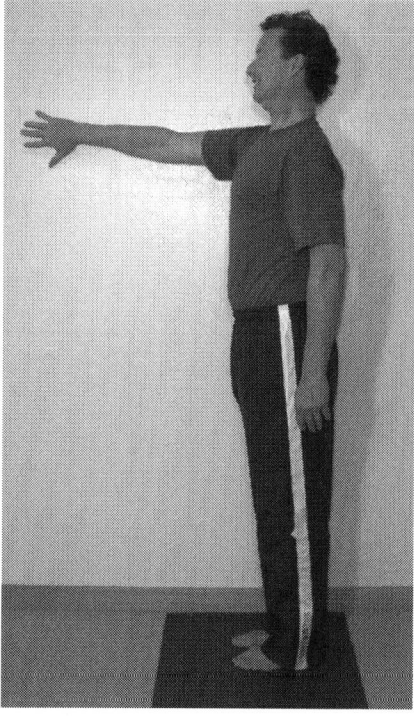

Arms behind interlace fingers and lift
Challenging

Stand with your legs right under your hips and feet pointing straight ahead. Pull up on your thighs (quadriceps). Be sure not to hyperextend your knees. Lift up through your spine. Lift the sides of your chest. Broaden through your top chest releasing the outside of your shoulders down towards your hips. Reach out through the crown of your head. Take your arms behind you and interlace your fingers with your wrists bent as shown in photo. Keeping your chest lifted, pull your arms back, lengthening through your arms and lift them up slightly. Take five to ten breaths and release.

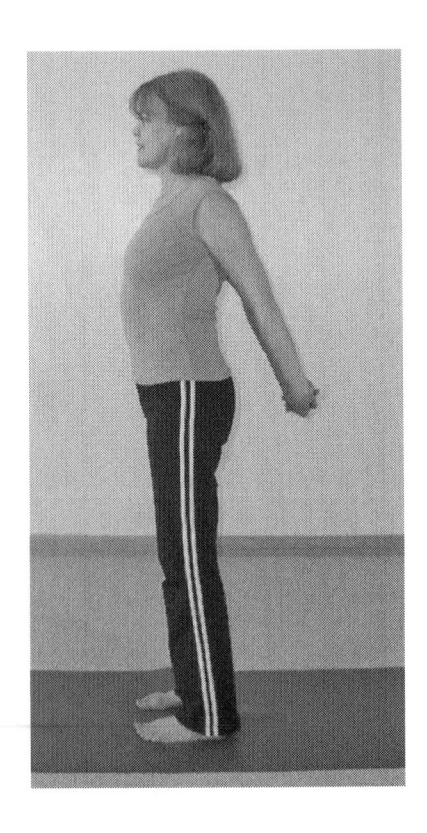

Eagle arms
Challenging

Stand with your legs right under your hips and feet pointing straight ahead. Lift up through your spine and broaden through your chest. Take both arms overhead towards the ceiling. Exhale and as you start to bring your arms down to the sides, bring them in front of your chest bending your elbows. Now place the left elbow inside of the right elbow crease (the space between your forearm and bicep). Turn your palms back towards each other and bring them together if possible. Don't worry if they don't touch. Lift your elbows up slightly and move them further in front of you so that you will feel more stretch through the backs and sides of your shoulders.

Note: This can be an intense exercise for some people. If it hurts in anyway, release a little or come out of it completely. Be sure to warm up with other exercises first.

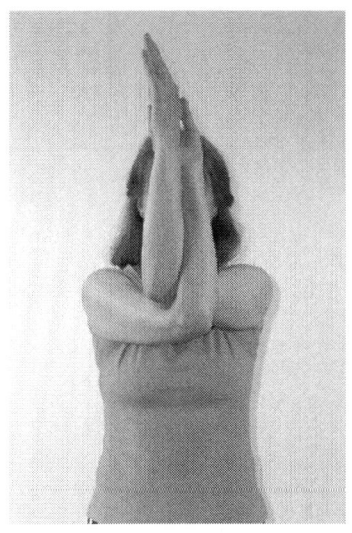

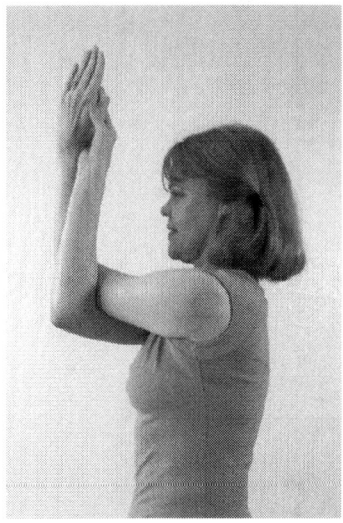

Downward facing dog with hands on block—3 ways
Challenging

The following versions of downward facing dog are great shoulder openers. However if you have weak wrists or wrist problems then go slowly. If these exercise hurt your wrists don't do them.

Place two yoga blocks on the floor and position them at an angle approximately 45% to the wall. Kneel on the floor and place your hands on the blocks with your middle finger pointing straight ahead. Walk your feet back so they are behind your hips, straightening your legs to come into downward facing dog pose (see page 32). Press your hands into the blocks and take your hips back. Take five to ten breaths. Come down and rest.

For the next version you will turn your hands in so that the fingers of one hand face the fingers of the other. Make sure your wrists are in line with your shoulders and step back into dog pose as indicated above. You may need to move the blocks a little closer. Take five to ten breaths. Come down and rest.

For the last version, turn your hands out, so that the fingers are facing away from each other. Be sure to have your wrists in line with your shoulders. You may need to move the blocks a little further apart. Take five to ten breaths. Come down and rest.

Note: These three variation work the shoulder muscles and joint in a different way each time you change your hand position. The result is a more open shoulder area. As a test of this take a regular dog pose on the floor before you begin using the blocks. After you use the blocks perform dog pose on the floor again and notice how different it feels.

65

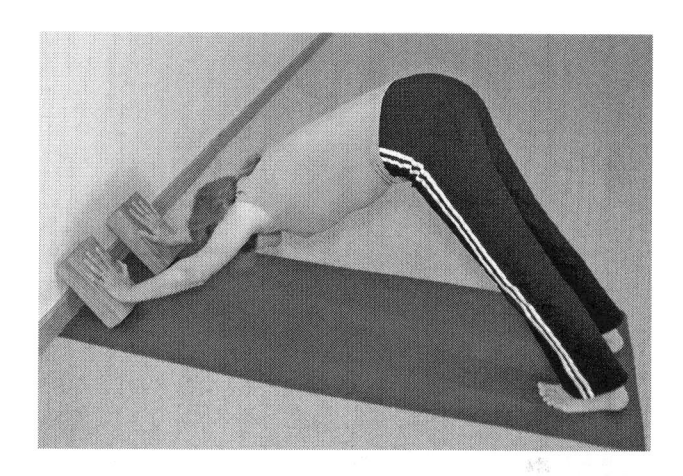

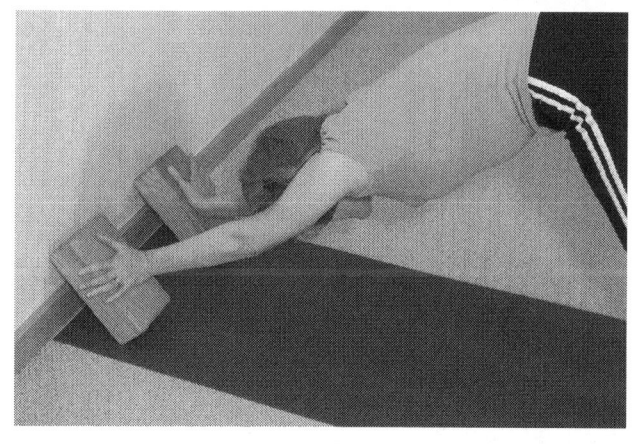

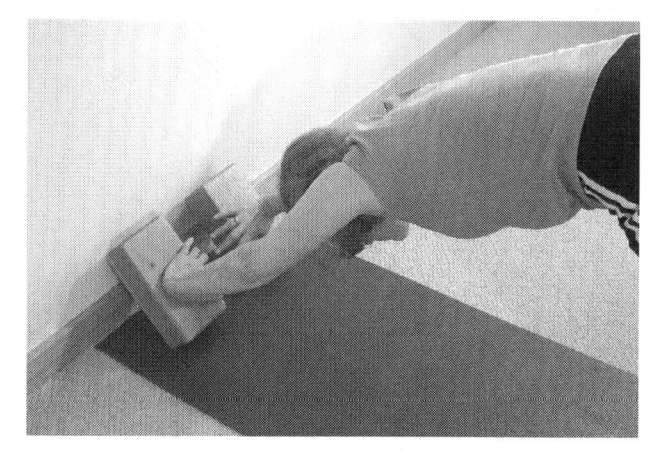

Triangle
Challenging

Take your legs wide apart—2 1/2 to 3 feet apart. Turn the toes of your left foot in slightly and from your right thigh turn your right foot out. Make you sure your right heel is in line with your left instep. Turn your hips to face forward. Stretch into your legs and lift up through your spine, broadening through your top chest. Take your arms to shoulder height and from the center of your chest extend through your arms. As you exhale, extend through your right arm and bend your torso sideways to the right. Be sure to keep your torso in line with your right leg—do not bend forward. Place your right hand on your shin or a yoga block. Press into your feet and extend through your legs. From your waist revolve your torso up towards the sky. Draw your shoulderblades away from your ears. Look up if you can—if it hurts to look up, look straight ahead or down at the floor. Press your right hand into your shin or the block and stretch your left hand away from that towards the sky. Take five to ten breaths. To come out, lift strongly through your left arm and inhale as you come up. Do the other side.

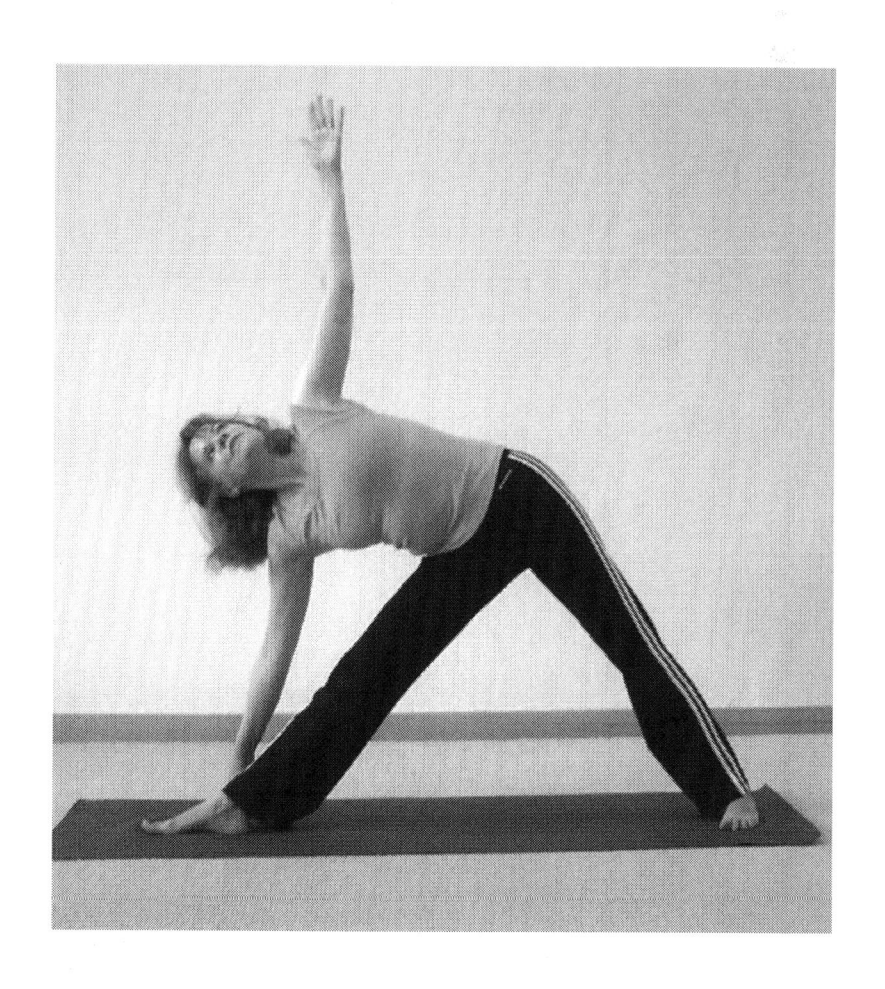

Warrior
Challenging

Step your right foot approximately 3 feet in front of your body. Turn your left foot in approximately 60%. Your hips should be almost square to your right leg so that your left hip is a little behind your right. Make sure your legs are in line with your hips. Lift up through your chest and take your arms overhead. Lift strongly through your arms as well as the sides of your chest and waist. Keeping the back foot on the floor, exhale and let your right knee float out over your right ankle. Take five to ten breaths and release your arms. Do the other side.

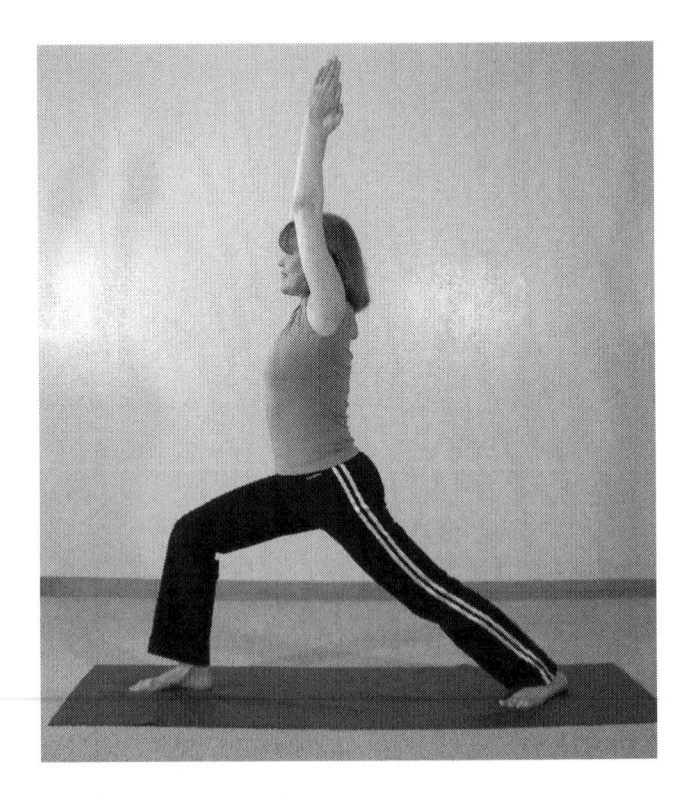

Grab forearm or elbow from behind
Challenging

Stand with your legs right under your hips and feet pointing straight ahead. Pull up on your thighs (quadriceps). Be sure not to hyperextend your knees. Lift up through your spine. Lift the sides of your chest. Broaden through your top chest releasing the outside of your shoulders down towards your hips. Reach out through the crown of your head. Take your hands behind you so that you grab the opposite forearm. If this feels easy grab the elbow instead. Let your arms nestle against your back. Lift your chest and draw your shoulder blades down. Be sure not to hyper-extend your lower back. Take five to ten breaths and release. Do this exercise again changing which hand is on top.

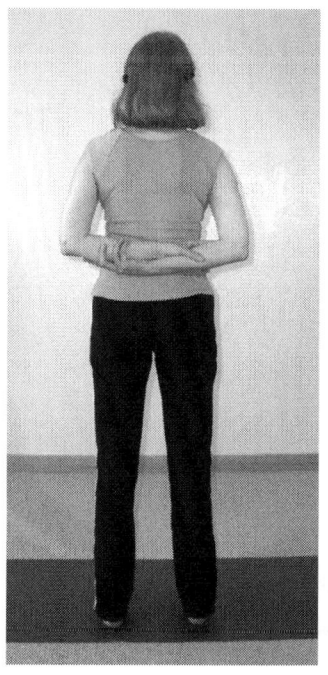

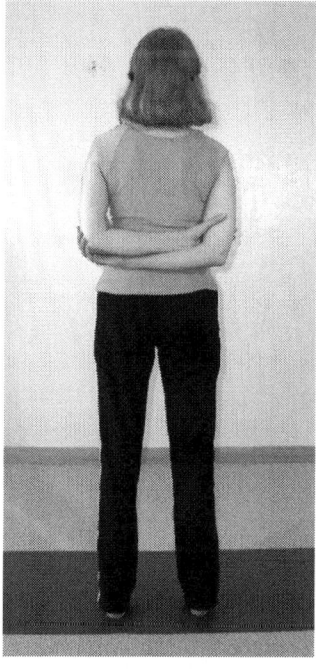

Strap work
Challenging

Stand with your legs right under your hips and feet pointing straight ahead. Lift up through your spine and broaden through your chest. Place a yoga belt or long piece of rope in your hands and take your hands about three feet apart. Bring your hands up overhead and reach up through your arms towards the ceiling. Take your arms back a couple of inches and continue to lift up. Take a couple of breaths here. Now, take your arms up and over so that your hands end up on the back of your body by your hips. Slowly take your arms back overhead to the front of your body.

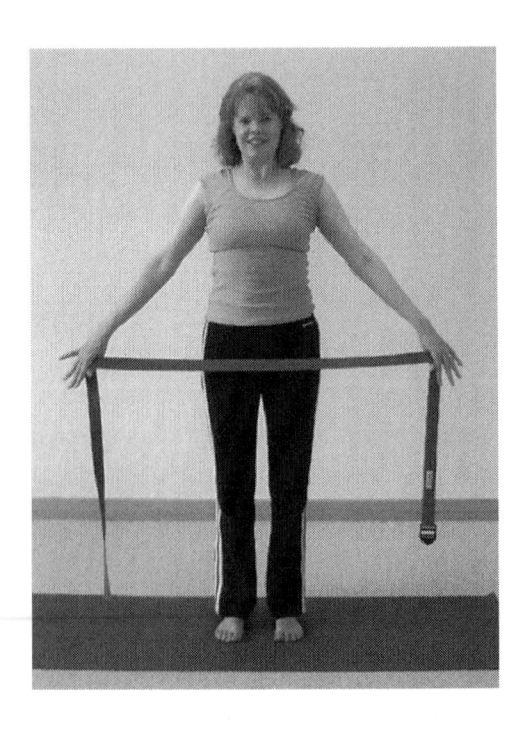

The secret to this exercise is having the strap the right length. It should offer a little resistance when you go up and over but not so much that you have to bend an elbow to get the strap over. Conversely it should not be too loose either as there will not be any resistance. Experiment with holding the strap in different places until you find the right resistance. Once you have the right width for your hands repeat the exercise three to five times. Pause after three times and take your hands in towards each other one half inch on each side and repeat the exercise.

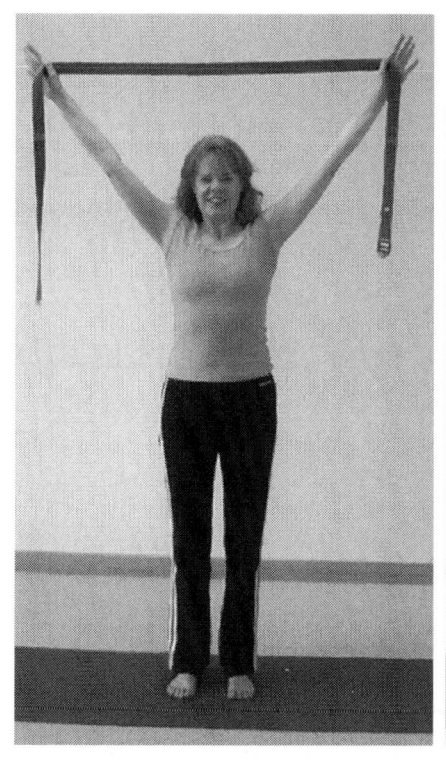

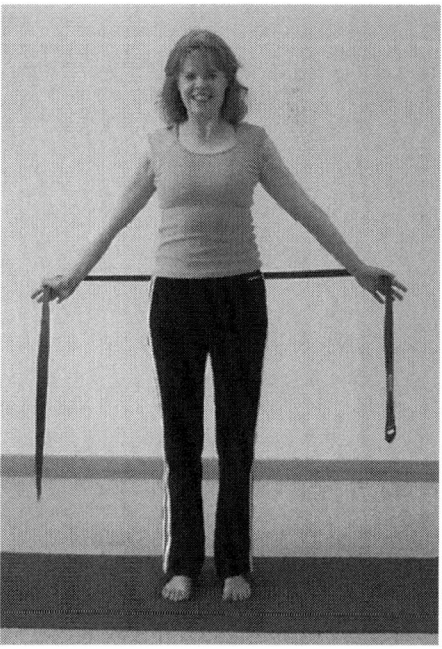

Cow's head pose
Challenging

This is a great posture but can be very intense—be gentle with yourself. Do this posture only after you have done many of the other exercises, especially the strap work on the prior page. If it hurts, ease up or don't do the posture. Remember, pain is an important signal from your body!

Stand with your legs right under your hips and feet pointing straight ahead. Lift up through your spine and broaden through your chest. Place a yoga belt (a strap, towel or old tie can work also) over your right shoulder. Extend your right arm up overhead and reach up towards the ceiling. Bend your right elbow placing your right hand on your upper back or lower neck and grab the strap. Take your left arm our to the left bending your elbow to allow your left hand to come onto your back grabbing the strap. Walk your right and left hand towards each other a little more if possible. Keep you chin parallel to the floor and be sure not to overarch your lower back. Take five breaths and release. Do the other side.

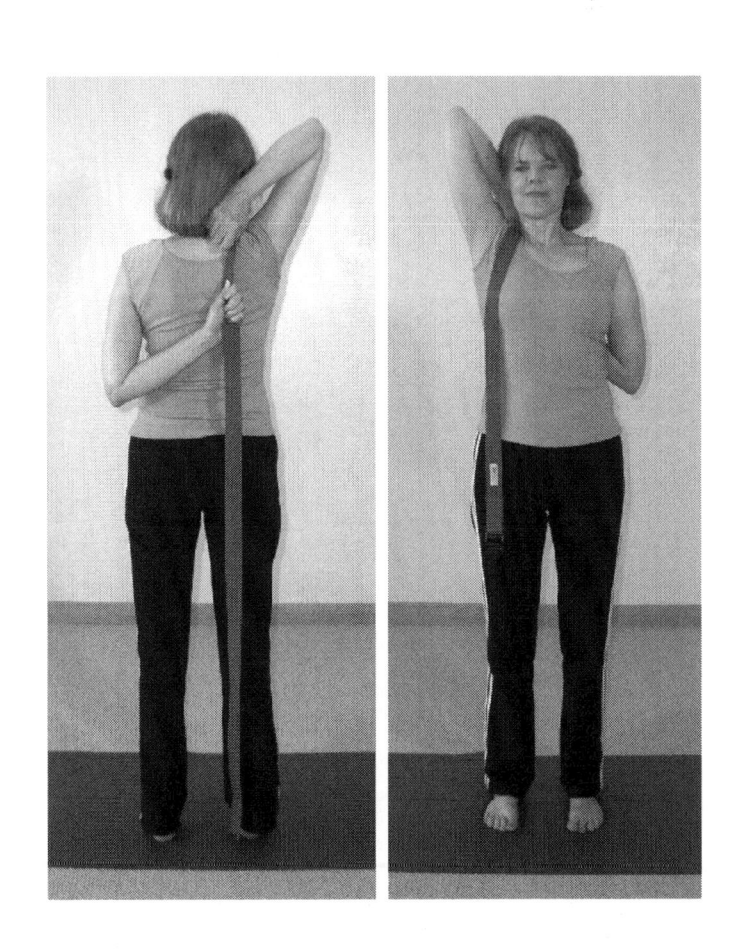

Sit on floor with hands behind— move forward

Challenging

This is a great exercise for stretching the front of the shoulders and the biceps. Sit on the floor and bend your knees, placing your feet on the floor. Take your hands behind you letting your torso go back slightly. Make sure your finger are facing away from you and your elbow are bent slightly. Lift up through your chest and extend your legs straight as shown in photo. Move your hips forward a couple of inches and notice how that increases the
intensity of the stretch. Take a few breath and then move forward again. Keep your chest lifted. Your can repeat this process a few more time but be sure to stop before it becomes too intense.

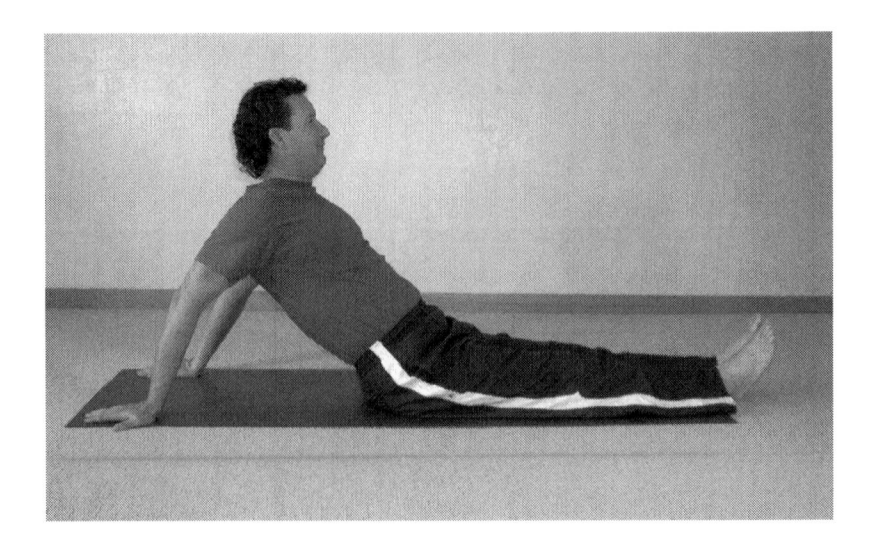

Hands pushing chair
Challenging

Place a chair in front of you as shown in the photo. Put a folded blanket approximately three feet in front of the chair. Lie on the floor face down, bringing your hips onto the center of the blanket. Extend your arms so that your palms are on the edge of the chair seat and extend through your fingers. Press your baby toes as well as your big toes into the floor. Stretch from your shoulders to your hands pushing the chair away from you. When you are fully extended allow your torso to relax. Take five to ten breaths and then carefully release to the floor. Rest here for a few breaths.

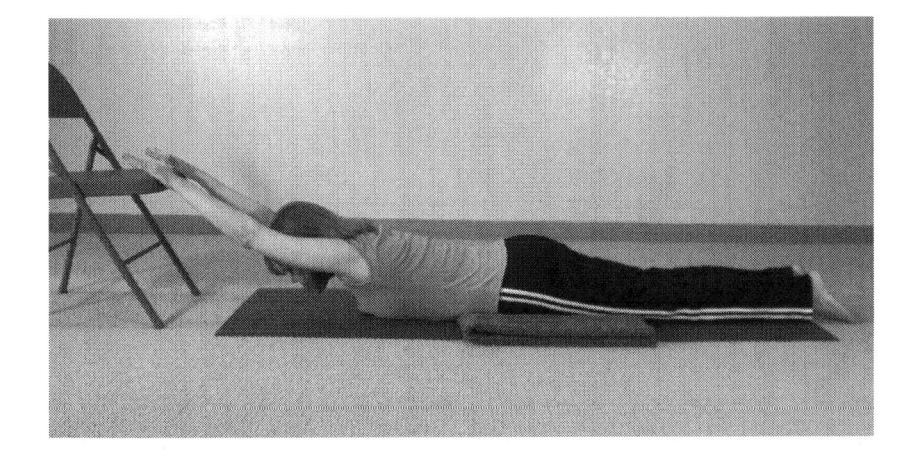

Locust (2 variations)
Challenging

Place a folded blanket on the floor as shown. Lie on the floor face down, bringing your hips onto the center of your blanket. Bring your chin or forehead onto the floor and your arms along side of your body with palms up. Bring your legs together or hip width apart. Make sure the baby toes as well as the big toes are pressing into the floor. Reach out through the crown of your head, draw your shoulders away from your ears and reach into your finger tips. From your inner thighs lift your legs and at the same time lift your torso, arms and palms up towards the ceiling. Broaden through your chest and lift more. Take five to ten breaths, come down and rest.

Here is a second variation of locust that helps to open the chest and the front of the shoulders even more. Laying on the floor face down bring your hands onto your hips and interlace your fingers so that your palms face the back of your head. Pull your hands away from your shoulders to pull your arms to draw the shoulders back. From the inner thighs lift your legs, torso and arms. Continue to use your hands to pull your arms drawing your shoulders away from your ears lifting your torso. Be careful not to pinch your inner shoulder blades together.

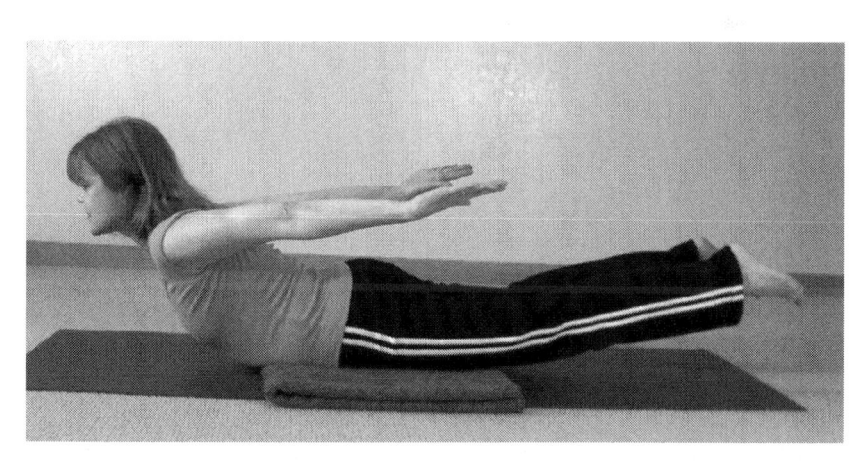

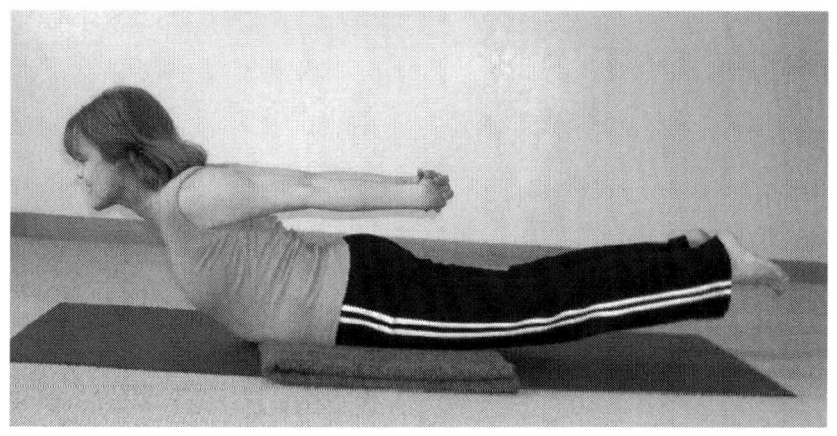

Bridge pose
Challenging

Lie on your back and bend your knees so that your feet are under your knees with your legs hip width apart. Extend your arms along the sides of your body. Press your feet into the floor and lift your hips and thighs off the ground. Walk your arms towards each other interlacing your fingers if possible. Keep extending through your arms, drawing your shoulders away from your ears. Press your arms and feet into the floor and lift your hips higher. Move your sacrum towards your pubic bone and take your hips higher. Move the base of your breastbone up and towards your chin to lift your chest even more. Take five to ten breaths and then release to the floor.

Note: Be careful of your lower back. If there is any compression come down a little or come out of the pose completely. Also, do not turn your head while in this position. Those with neck challenges should also proceed into this posture carefully.

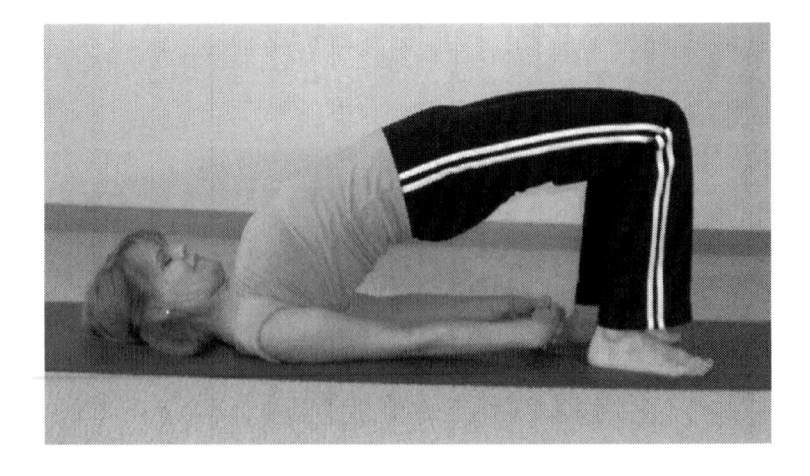

Gentle seated twist
Easy

Sit on a folded blanket as shown in the photo with your legs crossed. If you knees are higher than the tops of your hips sit on two blankets or even three if need be. Take your right hand to the outside of your left thigh and take your left hand behind you. Lift up through both sides of your chest and twist your torso more to your left. Broaden through your chest, collarbones and across the back of your shoulders. As you inhale lift up through your spine and as you exhale turn to your torso to your left a little more. Take five to ten breaths and release. Do the other side.

Note: The twists offer many benefits including stretching the deeper layers of muscles across your back and shoulders. They bring flexibility to the spine and stretch the muscles across the chest.

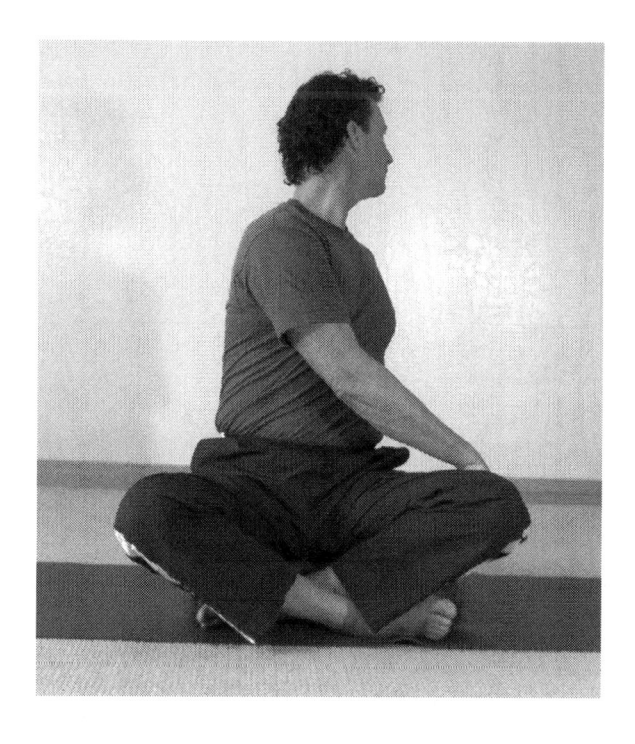

Half spinal twist
Challenging

Sit on a folded blanket. Bend your left knee so that your left foot is positioned by the outside of your right hip and your left knee is directly in front of you, more or less.

Bring your right foot over your left thigh and place it on the floor next to the front of your left thigh. Bring the elbow crease of your left arm around the top of your right shin and take your right hand behind you placing your finger tips on the floor. (If cradling your right shin in your left elbow crease feels like too much just place your hand on the outside of your right knee.) Turn to the right, broadening through your chest, collar bones and across your shoulders. As you inhale press your left leg into the floor and lift up through your spine, as you exhale twist a little more to the right.

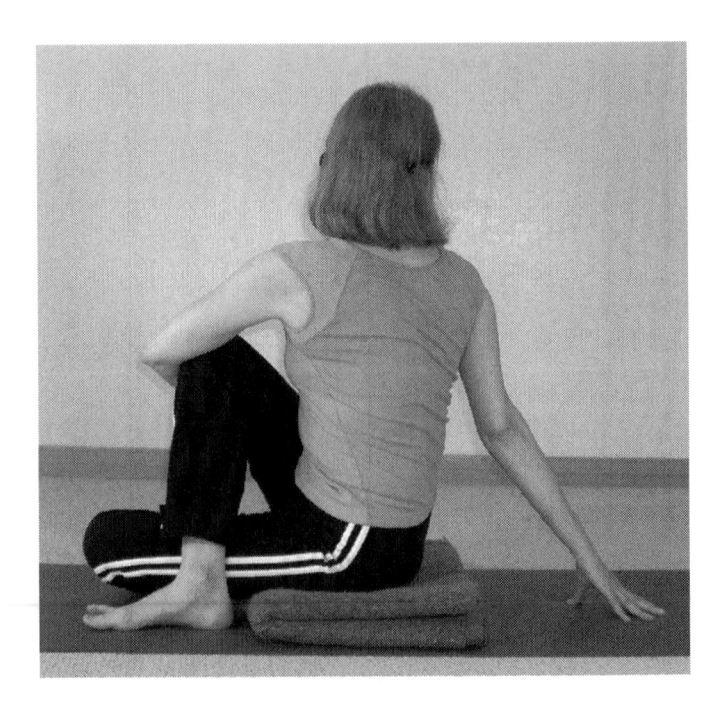

Tight Shoulder Relief Tip

Relax! Sometimes tight shoulders come from too much stress. If this is the case for you, it is important to find some ways to relax. Here are some suggestions: go for walk, exercise, do some yoga, engage in your favorite hobby, meditate, watch a funny movie, write in a journal, talk to a close trusted friend, plan a vacation.

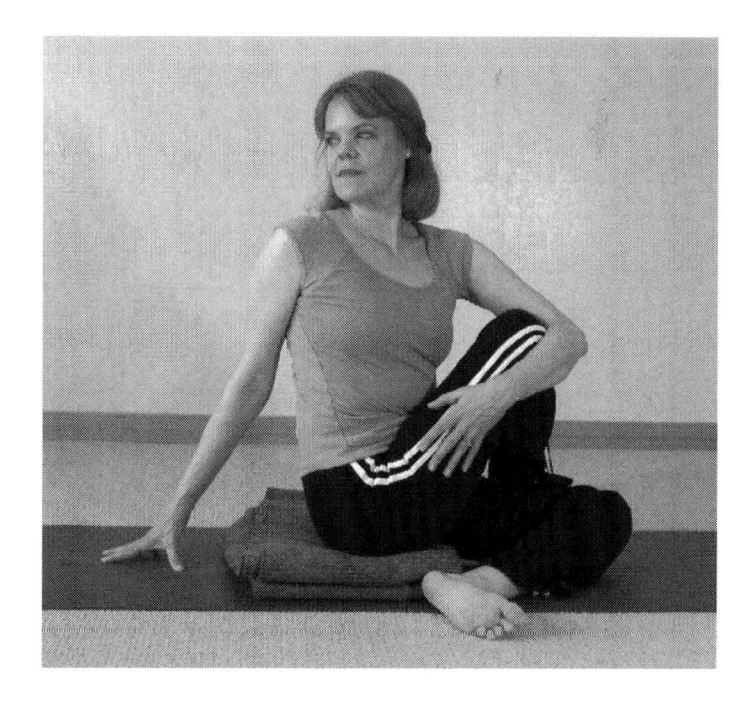

Seated elbow to knee twist
Challenging

Sit on a folded blanket with both legs extended. Bend your right knee and bring your right foot onto the floor in front of your buttocks. Let your left hip slide forward about two inches and move your right hip back slightly. Bring the fingertips of your right hand onto the floor behind your right hip. Take you left arm up overhead and bend your elbow bringing the triceps or elbow of your left arm to the outside of your right knee. Have your left hand pointing up towards the sky. (If bringing your left elbow over your knee feels like too much just use your left hand to hold the outside of your right knee.) Stretch into the left heel and keep your right leg centered—don't let it drop out to the right. As you exhale take your belly in and twist more to the right. Use your left arm against your right thigh as a resist to twist even more to the right. Broaden through your chest, collarbones and across your shoulders. Take five to ten breaths and then release. Do the other side.

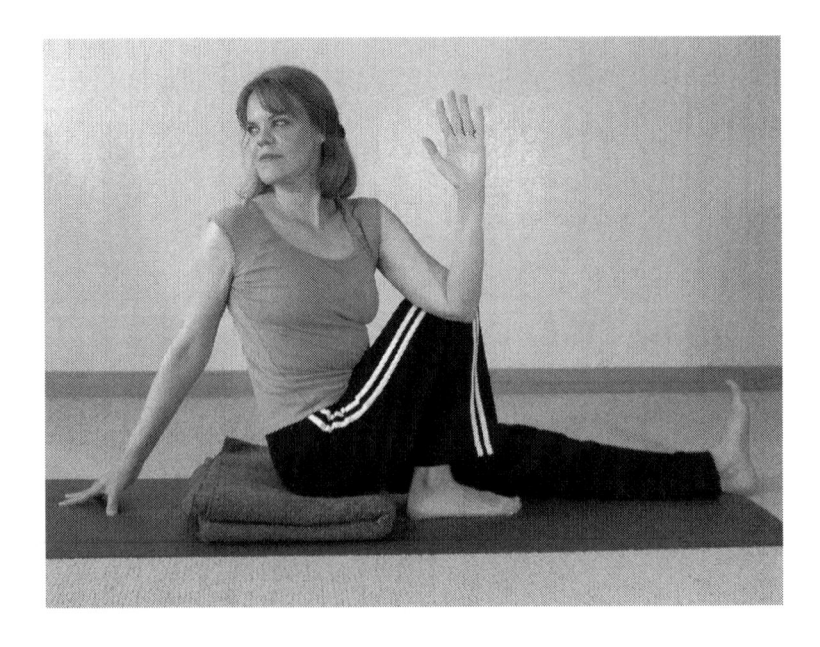

Knee down twist
Easy

Lie on your back. Extend your arms from your shoulders making a T position with your arms and torso. Move your hips a couple inches to the right. Bring your knees into your chest and then take them up and over to the left—to the floor. Look back to your right hand. Take 5 to 10 breaths and then repeat on the other side. For more challenge, extend your legs straight towards your hand once you are in the twist.

Note: Don't force your knees to the floor if they don't touch. Instead put something under your knees—such as a folded blanket, a pillow or some books.

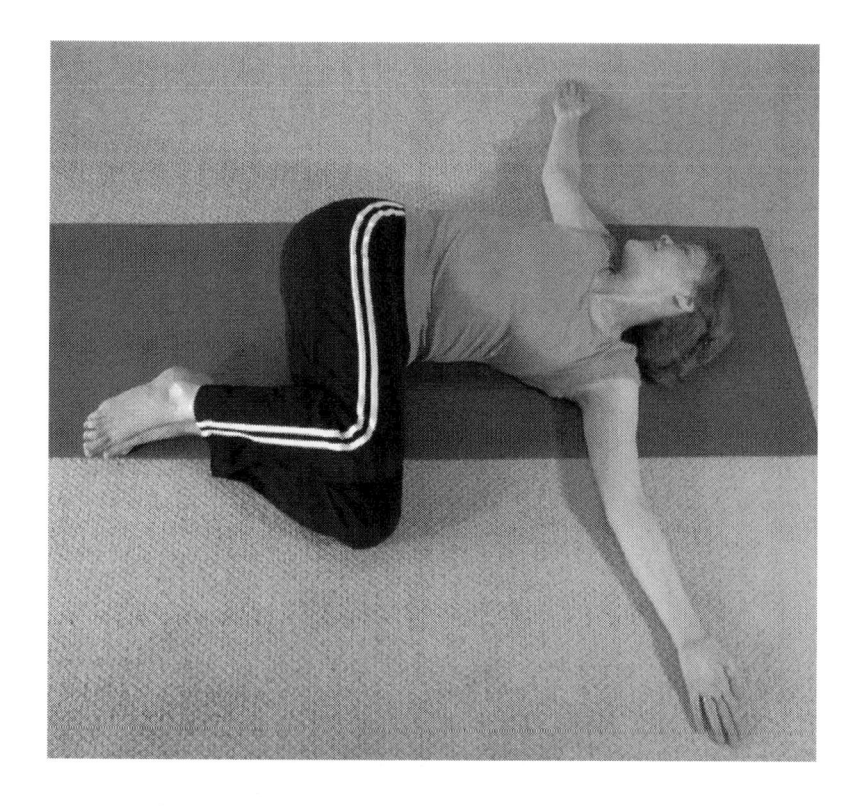

Foot on knee twist
Challenging

Lie on your back. Extend your arms from your shoulders making a T position with your arms and torso. Move your hips a couple of inches to the right. Place your right foot on your left knee. As you exhale take your right knee to the floor on the left side. Look back at your right hand. Start to take your right hand up overhead all the way to the left hand following with your eyes. Stretch through your left heel making your left leg long and firm your left hip. Keeping the right knee on the floor as long as possible take your right arm up overhead and back to the starting position following with your eyes. Your right knee may come off the ground—it is ok! Take five to ten breaths. Inhale to come up and do the other side.

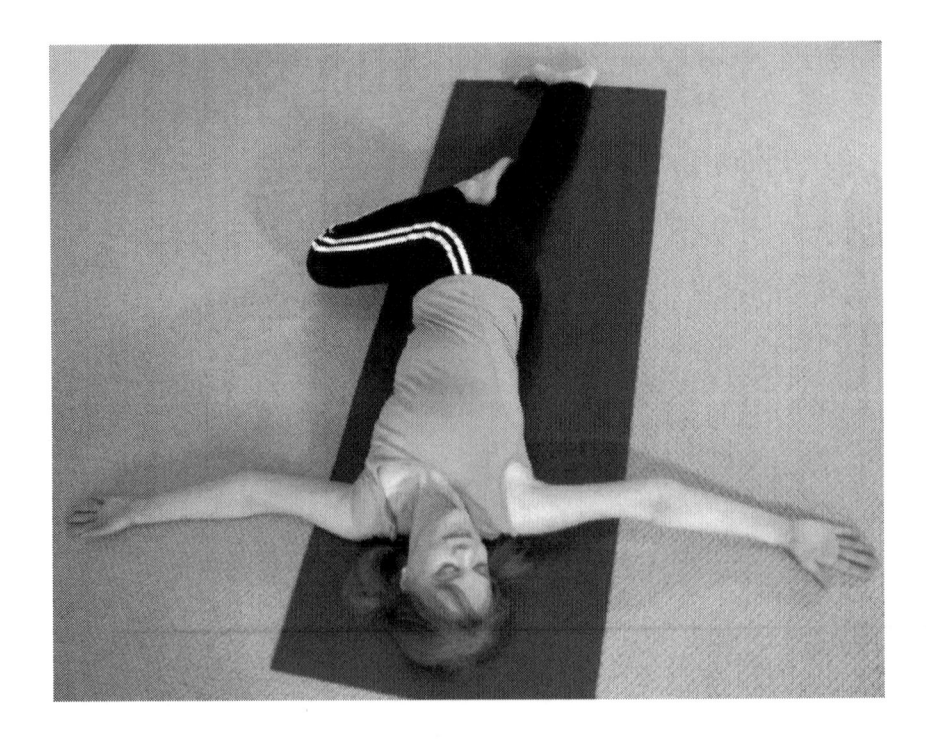

Additional ideas of interest

The following exercises require these props: yoga bolster, blanket, sandbags. I can already here some of you saying " I don't want to buy these things". These props are a very small investment in relationship to how much they can help you with your shoulders—you will find they are great gift to yourself and will last for many many years. Not only will they help bring great relief to your shoulders but you will also find they are deeply relaxing and restorative for your mind as well. For what you would spend at a nice restaurant for one good meal you can have the tools which will significantly impact the way you feel and how you go through life.

Chest opener over the bolster (1)
Easy

Set a round yoga bolster on the floor with a folded blanket placed over the bolster at one end. Sit at the other end (the end with no blanket) with your hips about six to ten inches away from the bolster. As you lean back have the end of the bolster meet your mid back, just under the tips of your shoulder blades. Place the blanket under your head and fold it again if you need more support for your head and neck. Let your arms drape to the floor at about 45% to your torso with the palms facing up. If needed, move the bolster forward or back a little until you feel comfortable. Ideally you should feel a good lift at the base of the breast bone. This is a great exercise for opening your chest and the front of your body and feels good too! Stay here for five to ten minutes.

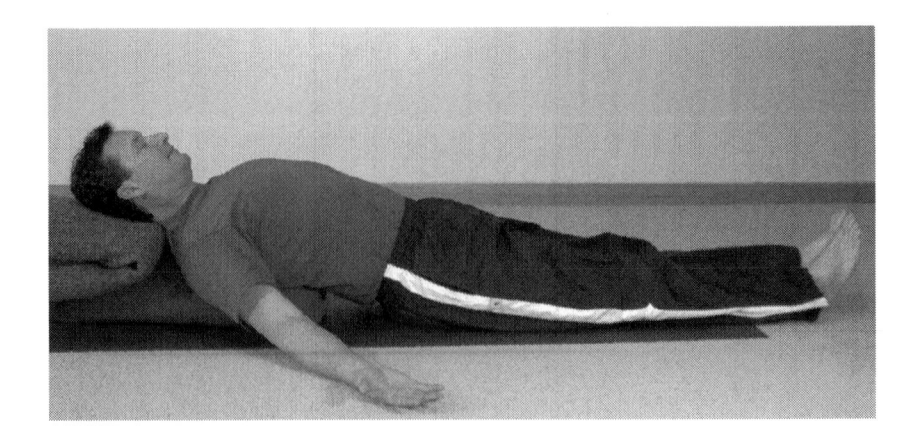

Chest opener over the bolster (2)
Easy

Place a round yoga bolster on the floor so that the width of it is facing your body when you sit down in front of it with your back facing the bolster. Place a yoga block or a couple of thick books just behind the back of the bolster. Lie onto the bolster so that you shoulder blades are on the bolster and your head rests on the block or books. Take you arms out to the sides at shoulder height. Your triceps should touch the back of the bolster. Make sure your head is supported well and there is no discomfort in your neck. Experiment with adjusting the height under your head up or down to see what feels best. Your legs should be extended straight in front of you. Take long slow breaths and stay here for five to seven minutes.

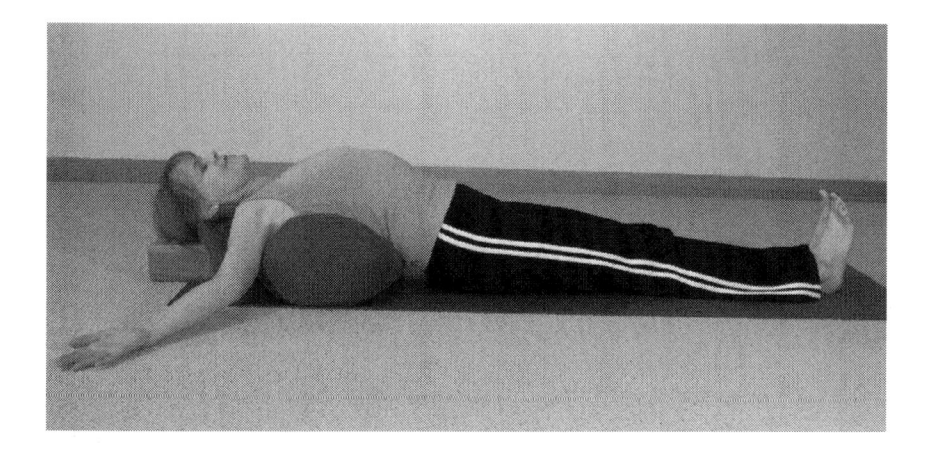

Sandbags on shoulders
Easy

Many people find this exercise feels terrific as well as therapeutic especially if there is a tendency to round the shoulders forward and collapse the chest. **On rare occasion using sandbags creates some discomfort—if this happens to you, don't do the exercise**.

Lie on the floor as shown with a folded blanket under your head. Make sure your legs, hips, torso, neck and head are all in one line. Allow your feet to drop to the sides. Place a ten pound sandbag across each shoulder so that part of the sandbag is resting on the shoulder and part of it is resting on the floor as shown in the photo. Take your arms to 45% with your palms facing up. Close your eyes and rest hear for five to ten minutes. To come out move the sand bags and slowly roll to your right side into a fetal position. Use both arms to slowly press up to a seated position.

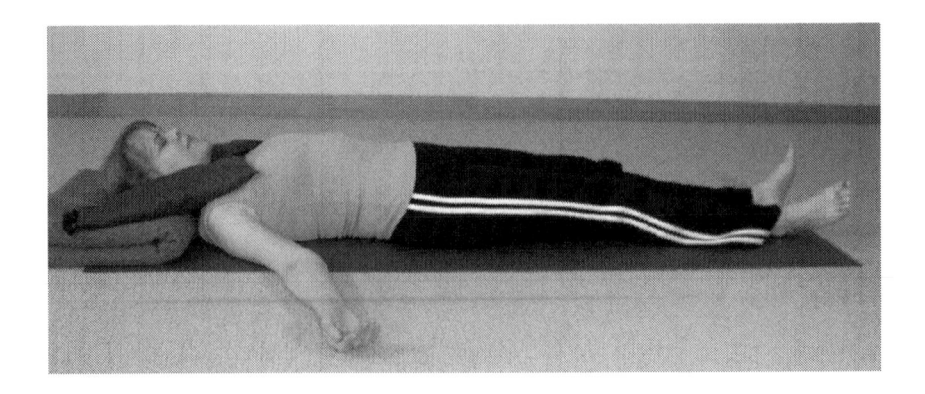

Tight Shoulder Relief Tip

Stop slouching! Sit up straight! You should have listened to your mother!

Kidding aside, when you slouch, your shoulders round forward and up—the trapezius and pectoral muscles tighten. Stay like this for any period of time and you get tight shoulders. When you catch yourself doing this remember to lift your collarbones up and draw your shoulderblades down your back and into your body. These simple movements will instantly transform your posture and the way you feel.

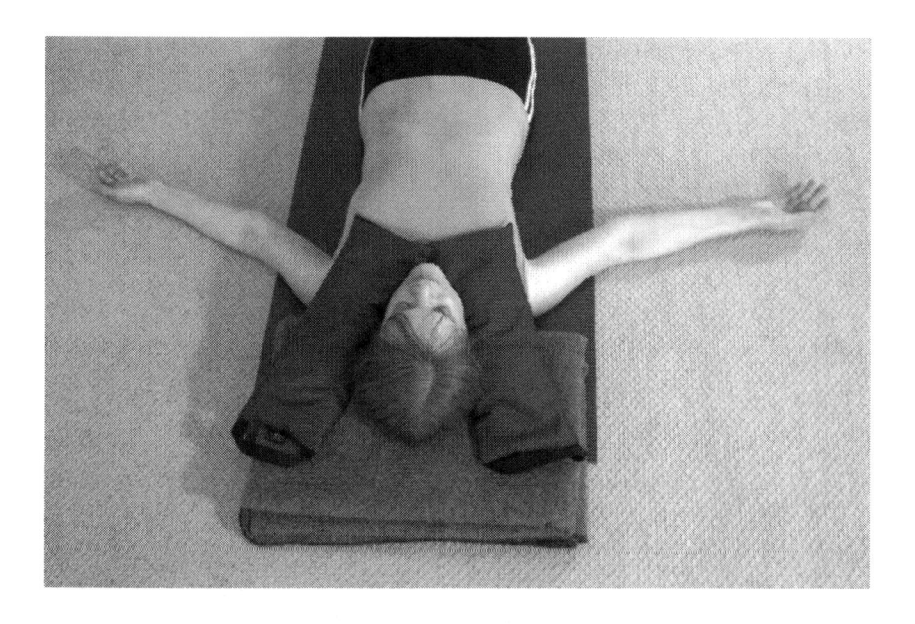

Chest opener over a blanket
Easy

Set a round yoga bolster on the floor, and center a yoga block or a couple of thick books on the floor behind the widest part of the bolster. Extend your arms out to the sides with your palms up. Rest here for a few minutes and then come to a seated position.

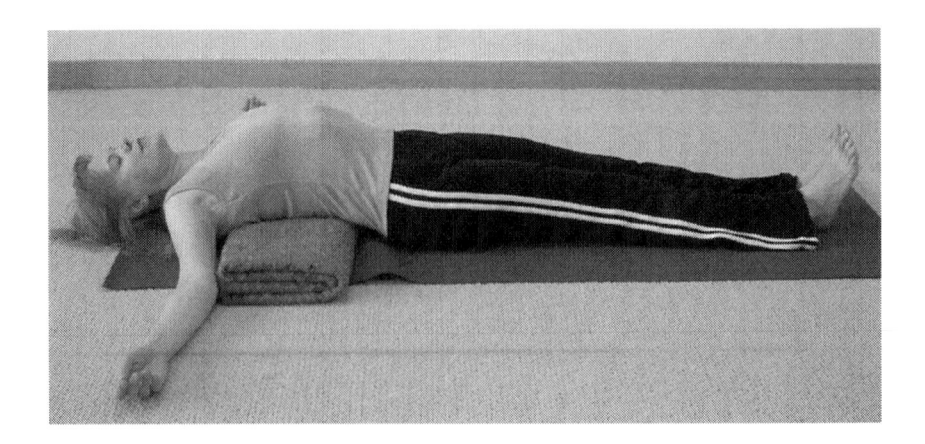

Also available from Letsdoyoga.com

On the following pages you will find additional wellness products and publications available from Letsdoyoga.com.

Additional books from Howard VanEs & Letsdoyoga.com

Beginning Yoga: A Practice Manual

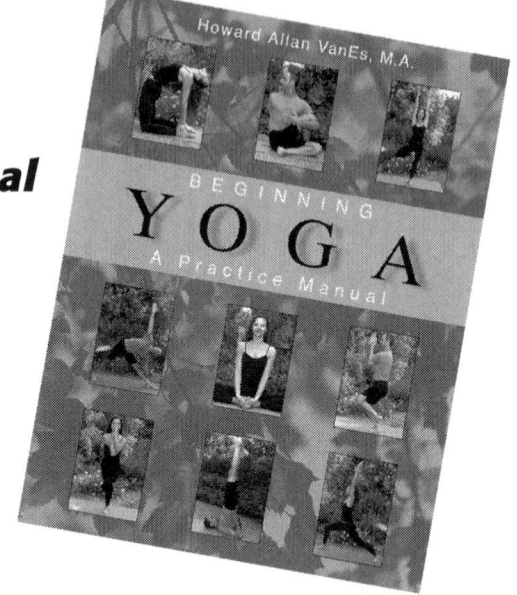

An essential resource for beginning through intermediate yoga students! *Beginning Yoga: A Practice Manual* has been carefully designed to help students develop a solid foundation in yoga through their home practice.

This is a clearly written, easy to use book with just the right amount of information to support your practice. And it's large 8 ½ X 11 format makes it easy to use. A thoughtful balance of theory and practice are presented to provide you with a context as well as instruction for your practice.

Features:

- Fifty postures detailed with full page photos and clear step-by-step instructions
- Intro to meditation
- Intro to pranayama (yogic breathing)
- Over 20 follow along practice sessions with words and pictures.
- Specific practices for energy, relaxation, and preventative back care.
- Lay flat book binding stays open for easy reference.

Visit www.letsdoyoga.com or www.amazon.com to order.

Office Ergonomics, Preventing Repetitive Motion Injuries & Carpal Tunnel Syndrome

By Susan Orr and Howard VanEs

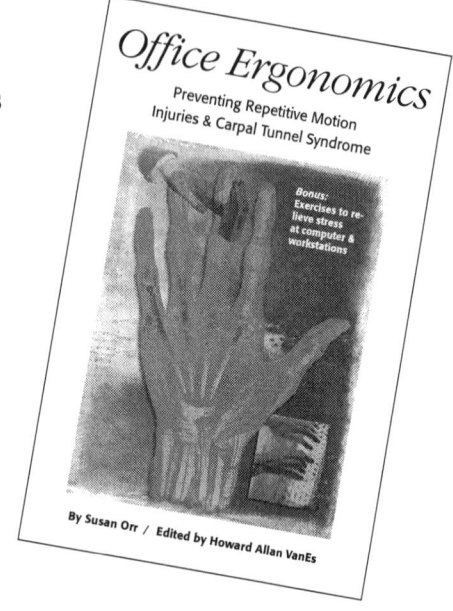

If your profession involves working at a computer or requires repetitive motion then the probability that you will experience an injury is very high.

Perhaps you are already experiencing symptoms such as tingling, pain, tightness or numbness in your wrist, elbow, shoulder, neck, or back. The good news is that there is a lot you can to do to prevent, eliminate, and reduce the possibility of injury.

Features: 100's of tips for making your workstation comfortable, efficient and for reducing the risk of injury. Causes and treatment of repetitive motion injuries. Positions and setups you must avoid. Fixes that don t work. Behavioral prevention tips. How ergonomics helps. Bonus: Exercises to relieve stress at computer & workstations.

Order at www.letsdoyoga.com or www.amazon.com

Ageless Beauty & Timeless Strength, A woman's guide to building upper body strength without any special equipment.

Learn how to dramatically reduce the risk of modern diseases and improve longevity without pills diets or creams.

Discover the life affirming benefits of body-weight exercises to: Lose weight while becoming stronger & more toned! Sleep better & become healthier overall! Experience more self - confidence and look & feel your best! Have more energy & enhanced sense of well-being!

Reverse osteoporosis: Strength training can stop the loss of bone AND increase bone bass by up to 9% within a year. Lose and maintain weight - stop yo-yo dieting. Reduce the risk of type 2 diabetes. Slow and prevent arthritis. Significantly reduce your risk of heart disease & high blood pressure. Could this be the fountain of youth? You decide!

Learn cutting edge nutrition secrets for maximizing strength & energy. Maximize your workouts to get the most benefits in the least amount of time. Fun, interesting, & challenging exercises for all levels.

Read inspiring biographies of women who use strength training to improve and positively impact their lives.

Order at www.agelessbeautybook.com and www.amazon.com

ABS! 50 of the best core exercises to strengthen, tone & flatten your belly.

Are you ready for a stronger, sleeker, slimmer belly?

Experience 50 of the very best ab and stomach exercises from Yoga, Pilates and other fitness modalities. They have been carefully selected for their effectiveness, ability to produce quick results and are fun to do. ABS! Goes well beyond old fashioned crunches and sit-ups.

Whether your belly is on the soft side or you're a high level athlete, you'll find a great variety of exercises that will target all four major groups of abdominal muscles, categorized by easy, moderate and challenging – so it is great for all levels of fitness.

This book doesn't make extreme promises like getting ripped abs in 6 days, doesn't recommend crazy diets that you're dying to get off of in a week, and there isn't a lot of technical mumbo-jumbo! When you purchase this book you will get highly effective ab and stomach exercises that will help you strengthen, tone and flatten your belly – in a healthy way.

Chapters include: 50 of the best ab exercises with photos and clear instructions, discussion of the many benefits of core exercises, overview of anatomy and more!

Available at www.amazon.com

Meditation: The Gift Inside

How to meditate to quiet your mind, find inner peace and lasting happiness.

What's it like to meditate? Imagine, for a moment, your mind chatter slowing - even stopping, if only briefly; you have clarity of mind and a feeling of expansiveness, creating a greater connection with yourself and the world around you. You experience a sense of peacefulness, wholeness and time can seem to stand still. Sounds good, doesn't it? It is!

For thousands of years mystics, ascetics, and everyday people have used meditation to draw them closer to the divine as well as for the numerous physical, mental, and emotional benefits of meditation.

These benefits include: reducing stress, sleeping better, lowering blood pressure, reducing pain in your body, enhancing mental focus and creativity, reducing anxiety and depression, improving your mood, and helps you live longer too.

In this book you will find powerful tools to transform your life. You'll discover what meditation really is, learn 7 time proven techniques, how make find. You'll get a little on the philosophy of yoga meditation, a section that discusses common challenges that people face in developing a meditation practice along with sound advice on overcoming them. You'll also learn how to deepen your meditation experience, suggestions for making it a regular practice and discover ways to bring meditation into your daily life.

Order at www.amazon.com

Printed in Great Britain
by Amazon